1996

CAPITATION FOR PHYSICIANS

Understanding and Negotiating Contracts to Maximize Reimbursement and Manage Financial Risk

CAPITATION FOR PHYSICIANS

Understanding and Negotiating Contracts to Maximize Reimbursement and Manage Financial Risk

JOHN F. MCCALLY

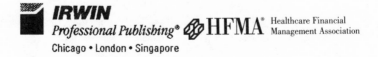

IRWIN
Professional Publishing® **HFMA** Healthcare Financial Management Association
Chicago • London • Singapore

Times Mirror
Higher Education Group

Library of Congress Cataloging-in-Publication Data

McCally, John F.

Capitation for physicians: understanding and negotiating contracts to maximize reimbursement and manage financial risk/John F. McCally.

p.   cm. — (HFMA management series)

Includes index.

ISBN 0-7863-1006-5

1. Managed care (Medical care)—United States. 2. Contracts. 3. Medicare. 4. Medicine—Practice. I. Title. II. Series.

RA413.5.U5M424   1996

362.1'0425—dc20   96–6446

Printed in the United States of America

1 2 3 4 5 6 7 8 9 0 BS 3 2 1 0 9 8 7 6

Dedication

This book is dedicated to those physicians, like my
friends Drs. Edward Rosenow III and Eugene Kern,
who have spent their careers helping their patients get
well, not only with excellent minds and a great deal of
technical competence but also with a personal healing touch.
For all such physicians, it is a pleasure to write a book
that can help you and your colleagues be successful in
this rapidly changing health care delivery environment,
so you can spend as much time as possible caring for
your patients.

I wish to thank many of my former colleagues,
including Jerry Wollner and Stan Salzman who have
helped me along the way, and particularly those whom
I have coauthored with like Stuart Lockman, Roger
Nauert, and Angie Miskowic. Last, but certainly not
least, I want to give my love, thanks, and appreciation
to my heavenly Father for His gifts to me including my
wonderful wife Elaine and my three outstanding
children, Lisa, Cray, and John, Jr., who have given me
years of love and support.

PREFACE

In today's managed care environment, successful physicians must constantly respond to change and plan for the future. When I started my health care career in 1959 with the Mayo Clinic, we had no computers in the business office; in fact, we were using the old punch card system. Today the combined clinics and hospitals of the Mayo system have more than 200 computer programmers assisting physicians and management with constantly changing data, as well as clinical and financial requirements to maintain quality care and cost efficiency. This is but a sample of where physicians find themselves today—in a state of perpetual transition. This transition is occurring in their everyday practice; clinically with rapidly changing technology, with definitely changing patient expectations, and potentially—even more dramatic—in the changing mode of reimbursement for the physicians' services.

Prior to joining the administrative staff of the Mayo Clinic, I was an economics major at Michigan State University. Little did I assume that basic economics would be a major force in the changes taking place in health care delivery today. However, we are in a major market transition, fueled by the underlying economic principles of supply and demand. The major factors of oversupply certainly include too many hospital beds, too many physicians, particularly too many specialty physicians in the more desirable locations in the United States. On the flip side of that economic theory, a limited amount of finances is available for third-party reimbursement (either by federal, state, or business payors) as well as a limited desire to regulate the apparent demand of the industry. This became very apparent in the summer of 1994 when the Democratic president and Democratic Congress could not pass a comprehensive reform bill.

Instead of comprehensive health care reform in the United States, we now have a marketplace where managed care is making major changes in the way health care is delivered and the way physicians are reimbursed. Even after physicians become contracted with managed care organizations (MCOs) change does not stop for each contract has a specific time period and often the contracts are changed as part of the renewal negotiation process. Because of that, many of the successful physicians, physician leaders, or practice and medical group administrators of the future will also become contract administrators.

As managed care enrollment continues to grow—currently at more than 10 percent per year—the number of patients being treated and the number of physicians under contract to treat those patients will continue to increase. Currently more than 150 million Americans are receiving care or are eligible to receive care from various managed care organizations, such as HMOs, PPOs, and POS plans. As physicians organize themselves into small single specialty groups, larger multispecialty groups, or medical foundations and develop various methods to maintain a more competitive nature in the health care marketplace today, these new organizations and their physician leaders find themselves in the category of multimillion dollar businesses. Indeed, two of the organizations where I was in administration, the Mayo Clinic and the Detroit Medical Center, now have gross revenues exceeding $1 billion a year. Having worked as a national consultant for two national accounting and consulting firms where I also assisted many medical groups, multispecialty physician clinics, and network organizations, I can indicate from experience that the former cottage-industry organizations in health care are today multimillion dollar businesses. As such they need to plan and implement changes appropriate for million dollar businesses, in a $1 trillion a year industry.

The purpose and direction of this book is to assist physicians, their leadership, or their financial advisors and consultants in how best to not only survive but also be successful in today's changing managed care and capitation environment. As I have lectured to physicians and financial advisors across the country, many have been surprised when I have stated up front that current medical practices can be financially successful under managed care and capitation. However, achieving success takes an understanding of the changes in the health care industry, particularly with changing reimbursement and its impact on practice patterns and incentives. And as I'll stress in the chapters following the sample capitated contract, the financial success of a physician's practice in the future will not depend on just good negotiation. It will be imperative that the implementation of the contract in the physician's office be done in a cost effective manner. For those physicians and administrators who read this book searching for answers, I strongly recommend that you not only understand these concepts and recommendations but also recognize that managed care organizations, contracts, and reimbursement will change dramatically from one medical service area to another and from one year to the next. Therefore, please realize that there is no one answer now or in the future to being successful under managed care and capitation. This ongoing process takes thorough understanding, flexibility, planning, and a commitment to change, to truly be successful. Having seen positive results of such change, I know it can be done. I wish you all the best in improving your profits through managed capitation.

CONTENTS

Chapter 1

The Changing Dynamics of Health Care Reimbursement   1

Chapter 2

The Changing Organizational Dynamics of Physician Practices   9

Success through Change   11
The Growth of Group Practices   13
The Move to Integrated Systems and Relationships   16

Chapter 3

The Stages of Managed Care Development and Their Impact on Physicians   21

Shifting Financial Risk   21
Five Stages of Managed Care Evolution   23

Chapter 4

Models for Physician Responses and Managed Care Participants   27

Staff Model HMO   27
Group Model HMO   29
Network Model HMO   29
Independent Practice or Physician Association (IPA) Model HMO   30
Preferred Provider Organization (PPO) Model   31

Chapter 5

Major Contract Issues That Impact Physicians in Managed Care Contracts   33

Chapter 6

Analyze Your Current Practice Activity before Looking at a Contract 41

Practice Actively Analysis 42

Analysis of Impact of Potential Managed Care System Participation 47

Chapter 7

Fifty Questions to Improve Your Bottom Line and Negotiation Strategy 51

Chapter 8

Analysis and Review of Sample Capitated and Medicare Contracts 57

Sample Contracts 58

Questions Relating to the Capitated Contract Example 95

Chapter 9

Analytical Process for Calculating Capitated/Risk Contract Rates 103

Analytical Process for Calculating Risk Contract PMPM Rates 104

Step 1: Define All Services Included in the Capitation Contract 105

Step 2: Risk Adjust Medical Services 106

Step 3: Identify All Other Variables Included in the PMPM Premium Rate Model of the Health Plan or Direct Contractor 108

Step 4: Adjust for Current HMO/Health Plan Demographic Factors 108

Key Managed Care Performance Indicators 115

Provider Incentives and Rewards 117

Chapter 10

How to Develop a Managed Care Strategy: Remember You Only Get What You Negotiate 119

Practice Strategic Analysis 120

Financial Risk Assessment 122

Counterproposal Preparation 124

Chapter 11

Recognizing the Change and Impact of Going from Discounted
Fee-for-Service Contracts to Capitation   127

Chapter 12

Physician Income Distribution Systems under Capitation   137

Chapter 13

Management Information Systems Improve the Chances for
Success of a Capitated Contract   147

Chapter 14

The Benefits of Using Cost Information When Implementing
Capitated Contracts   155

Chapter 15

Legal Concerns and Issues in the Managed Care/Capitated
Health Care Delivery System   161

Appendix: Managed Care Resources and Organizations   169

Glossary   173

Index   194

1

CHAPTER

The Changing Dynamics of Health Care Reimbursement

To begin, recall that health care reimbursement was basically 100 percent fee-for-service until the 1930s. At that time, two things happened from a health care insurance reimbursement standpoint that have had significant impact on physicians and their practice of medicine some 60 years later. The first event was the original capitation paid by the Kaiser Corporation for the health care of their employees on the West Coast. Kaiser, which at that time was making aluminum and steel, decided that their employees needed to be taken care of on a regular basis by competent physicians. They started that care by hiring physicians who were paid five cents per month for each of the Kaiser employees at a plant. The second event occurred at approximately the same time. Several states started discussing, then licensing and approving businesses that sold health insurance to employers for their employees, as well as to individual citizens.

With the advent of World War II, health insurance was hardly a priority issue. However, following World War II, many employers anxious to hire former soldiers and sailors started buying the more traditional indemnity insurance for their employees. As employees became more and more unionized during the late 1940s and early 1950s, unions started making health insurance part of their contract negotiations with employers. This created a major surge in the growth of what we consider the old system of traditional, fee-for-service medical insurance. Such insurance gave the patients greater flexibility and provided employers with a range of contract options they could offer to their employees.

Under most fee-for-service, indemnity insurance plans, physicians practiced medicine with considerable freedom of choice about practice matters and medicines; meanwhile, patients had similar freedom to choose which physicians they would go to for their problems. The majority of physicians in the 1940s, 1950s, and 1960s were paid by their patients directly or they had relatively few problems getting reimbursed from indemnity insurance companies on submission of appropriate claims. Often times, the biggest problem for physicians in the 1950s and 1960s was the multitude of different claim forms and different reimbursement procedures created by a rapidly growing proliferation of health care insurance companies. Such reimbursement trends have not continued with the growth of managed care and its impact on physicians.

Today, managed care and HMOs often are used interchangeably. However, there is truly a significant difference from many aspects, including both reimbursement for physician services and control over what and how a physician provides that care. I explore the difference between managed care and HMOs in the later chapters of this book. At this point it is important to clarify the overall concept of managed care. The following definition of managed care is from the Health Insurance Association of America:

> A system, plan, or organization *integrating* the financing and delivery of *appropriate* health care services to covered individuals using the following basic elements:
>
> ♦ *Significant financial incentives* to use providers and procedures *associated* with the plan.
>
> ♦ *Formal programs* for *ongoing* quality assurance and utilization review.
>
> ♦ *Explicit standards* for the selection of health care providers.

Just a quick definition as a follow-up to the first element in the preceding paragraph; an HMO (health maintenance organization) could be what is referred to there as *the plan*. There are multiple managed care organizational models that offer multiple plans to various employers. Later chapters go into detail about the multiple contracts for different health care providers. The most common managed care organizations today are the HMOs, PPOs (Preferred Provider Organizations), and POS (Point-Of-Service) plans.

Note that the definition from the Health Insurance Association of America contains several key words that must be understood by those physicians, and their administrators, who are currently becoming more involved or involved for the first time with a managed care organization. Those key phrases include from the opening paragraph the word *appropriate,* and in the first element, the word *incentives.* Also in the first element, the word *associated.* In the second element, the word *ongoing,* and in the third element, the word *standards.* All of these key words can have a significant impact on physicians, their office activities, their patient load, and the types of services they provide to patients. Perhaps even more important, their office activities and the reimbursement of physicians may be based on the measurement of physician services by an ongoing program that meets certain standards, all set potentially by someone other than the physicians who control or care for the patients.

Certainly in the 1950s and 1960s, the previous information about managed care was not of concern to the majority of physicians. Today managed care has become the dominant mode of health care delivery in the United States and providers are expected to deliver not only on price but also on value, quality, and performance. Managed care has grown in the last 20 years; now more than 150 million Americans are receiving their care through managed care companies and programs. This does not include the rapidly growing movement in both Medicare and Medicaid of having enrollees receive care through a managed care program.

What is creating this rapidly changing health care delivery environment? *The marketplace is driving health care change today. This has created a state of perpetual transition for providers.* As the health care reform debate created news stories, articles, books, and television commercials in 1993 and 1994, it also created a strong awareness of what is happening in the health care delivery marketplace.

As experts forecast, the health care industry has now arrived and become a $1 trillion a year industry. State governments have found their budgets for Medicaid spending averaging 18 percent of their total budgets, up from 10 percent only five or six years earlier. The federal government is spending billions on Medicare with no leveling off in sight. Now, a year after health care reform efforts in Congress were declared dead, we hear from both parties that Medicare will be broke within a relatively short time if the system does not get changed. Congress is discussing a number of alternatives for that kind of change. Many alternatives are rooted in the Health Security Act President Clinton proposed in 1993; that is, some type of managed competition or managed care.

Currently a number of states already have Medicare HMO enrollment. Arizona and California, for example, have 28 percent of their Medicare population enrolled in a managed care plan. (See Figure 1–1.)

The most compelling reason that the health care marketplace is and will continue to be in a state of perpetual transition, however, is the cost to U.S. employers of providing health care benefits to their employees. Although this figure varies from region to region and state to state, in 1994 U.S. employers paid an average of $3,741 per employee for health care benefits according to a national survey of employer-sponsored health plans by Foster Higgins & Co., Inc., in 1995. Note that the Midwest had the highest average in 1994, with $4,048 per employee whereas the South was the lowest with $3,389 per employee. Currently, the dynamics of managed care often reflect the size of the marketplace, the supply of the physicians (i.e., the potential oversupply of certain specialties or the oversupply of hospital beds), and the number and type of managed care plans in that marketplace. As an example, Minneapolis has a very high number of HMO plans and is fairly similar to Boston. However, Minneapolis has more PPO plans than HMO plans, whereas Boston has relatively few PPO plans, thus creating different managed care dynamics.

The impact of the differences of HMO and PPO penetration in a given marketplace, compared to another given marketplace, also depend on the types of contracts negotiated between those various managed care companies and the health care providers or organizations. Such organizations could include solo practitioners in an IPA (independent practice/physician association) type of

FIGURE 1–1

Medicare HMO Enrollment 1990–94
(top 10 states)

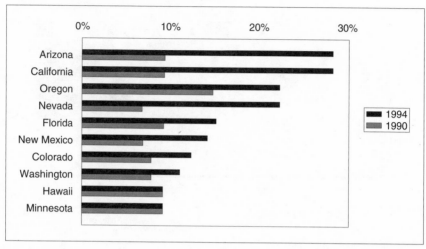

Source: Health Care Financing Administration

HMO or groups in a PHO (physician hospital organization), specifically put together to *negotiate managed care contracts and accept the financial risk of capitation.*

The previous sentence indicates the key underlying difference between the old, indemnity type of health insurance and the rapidly growing, dominant mode of health care delivery today, managed care; that is, the shift in whole, or part, of the financial risk for the cost of providing services to a patient or group of patients to the providers of that care. (See Figures 1–2 and 1–3 that explain the difference to the provider of the change between fee-for-service reimbursement and capitation to be explained in greater details in Chapters 8–11.)

The ever-changing marketplace has continued to put pressure on managed care companies to reduce premium costs to employers. This has resulted in more managed care companies turning to capitation as a way to not only shift financial risk to providers but also change physician and hospital incentives, as discussed in a later chapter. A second major mechanism to reduce cost and shift risk that we also discuss in a later chapter is direct contracted care.

FIGURE 1–2

Fee for Service Medicine
(*Volume + Revenue = Profit*)

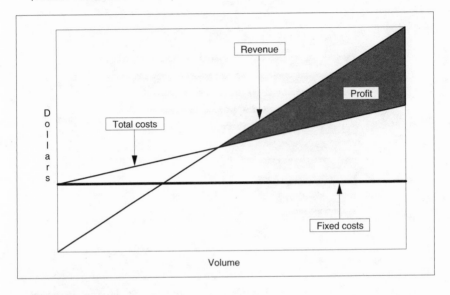

FIGURE 1–3

Capitated Medicine
(*Revenue–Costs = Profit Volume + Costs = Loss*)

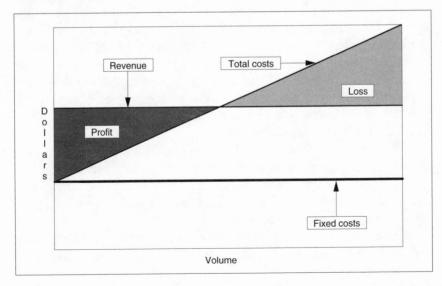

Figure 1–4

The Changing Paradigm of Health Care Cost Reduction Activities

1980s	1990s
Second opinions	Protocols
Controlled length of stay	Fixed payments
Physician credentials	Physician profiles
Large panels and networks	Target providers
Comprehensive cost coverage	Copays and deductibles
Service menus	Packaged programs
Fee arrangements	Capitation
Managed care	Direct contracted care

Any mention of contracted care brings to mind a series of evolutionary changes in health care delivery and reimbursement over the last 10 to 20 years. Figure 1–4 on the changing paradigm of health care cost reduction activities lists the major changes in activities during the 80s and 90s. 'As you can see from the chart, the last line refers to the changes in the 1990s that we are seeing where reimbursement is changed from managed care to direct contracted care.

Capitation may be used under both managed care and direct contracted care as a way of reimbursing physicians and other health care providers, as well as a way for the third-party payors to control their health care costs. For the purposes of this chapter, we refer to direct contracted care as that growing movement across the United States where either large employers or groups of employers such as business coalitions, organized their employee benefit programs so that they can contract directly with the physicians, hospitals, and other providers necessary to provide care at a predetermined rate. Another trend emerging from direct contracting is that often contracts are for longer than one year. In effect, the physicians and/or other signers of direct contracted care contracts are accepting the risk financially for the care of a set number of employees for a set amount of reimbursement. In certain cases, this approach by employers or business coalitions eliminates the average administrative overhead fee of 12 to 18 percent of most managed care organizations. In reality, the managed care companies carry out marketing, underwriting, and contracting functions that do not go away but are often taken on by either the employers or the providers themselves.

Let us always remember that many managed care organizations are in business to make a profit. Often times they have been successful by keeping as much as possible of the employee premium paid by the employer. They do this through negotiating contracts with health care providers. My experience has been that those providers who are most successful in this environment—that is contracting with a managed care company or a business coalition—and others who will be successful in the future, coordinate the care of their patients on an integrated basis with other health care providers, while at the same time have access to experienced health care business and contract advisors. Physician organizations in the 1990s are definitely $1 million, $5 million, $10 million, $50 million, or $100 million a year and more businesses. To be successful in the contracted world of health care delivery in the future, providers need to be organized so that they can not only accept financial risk through capitation but also implement managed care contracts on a daily basis in a businesslike manner. They can do this by knowing and evaluating their costs of providing that care, while at all times recognizing the importance of continuing to provide appropriate and measurable, quality care.

Having brought to the forefront the subject of provider integration, this becomes a very appropriate place to talk about the various physician responses that have developed over the last 20 years as mechanisms to provide cost effective, quality medicine, particularly in managed care environments. This leads to our next chapter, The Changing Organizational Dynamics of Physician Practices.

2 CHAPTER

The Changing Organizational Dynamics of Physician Practices

"Economics is a subject that does not greatly respect one's wishes."

Nikita S. Khrushchev

Physician responses to the rapidly changing environment have taken many different forms over the past two decades. From forming single specialty groups through developing vertically integrated delivery systems, physicians have changed their organizational structure. Some physicians have decided that as independent or solo physicians they truly will be at a disadvantage in dealing with insurance companies and managed care plans. Other solo practitioners have simply been overwhelmed by the ever-increasing paperwork and regulations federal and state governments have created, to say nothing of the multiple requirements from multiple insurance companies. The best example of that came to me when as the administrator for a large, multispecialty clinic in Detroit at the end of the 1980s, I found that our front desk personnel, business office personnel, and physicians, all needed to be aware of and follow different procedures and protocols for more than 100 insurance companies and managed care plans.

Depending on the part of the country, many solo physicians today also are seeing patients leaving their practice to go to larger, newer, or integrated group practices as well as HMO clinics. In addition, as physicians often finish their residency owing thousands of dollars in bank loans for their medical school training, it makes economic sense to join a group practice or an HMO that is already established and where someone else takes care of administrative details so the physician can practice medicine while earning a set salary each month. When joining medical groups, or merging their practice with others, physicians who have been in private practice often find that economically they have gained economies of scale. As such they can afford the business office expertise/consultants to assist them with managed care contracting and other pertinent business decisions as physician practices collectively become million or multimillion-dollar-a-year businesses. Certainly, in larger metropolitan areas where 25 percent or more of the marketplace is controlled by in managed care plans, it becomes a defensive mechanism for physicians to leave the solo practitioner environment. They can then be part of a physician group or organization that can compete for patients, as opposed to the solo physician who no longer gets certain patients because he or she is not a member of a particular physician "panel" serving a given managed care plan.

As the insurance and managed care companies have grown over the last two decades, so has the need for providers to have appropriate management information to work with and use to talk to the insurance company/managed care plans. There are still occasional solo physicians who do not have computer systems. However, the requirements of providing information to Medicare, Medicaid, insurance companies, managed care plans and often state governments, now make managed information systems an essential part of the physician's business. Once again for many physicians this type of change has created the need to make a decision to leave solo practice and join some other type of larger physician organization. In some service areas, managed information systems are necessary to provide the data to be used to market physician services, usually for medical groups and physician organizations, based on measurable quality care and outcomes of that care, not the old marketing criteria of convenient and quality physicians. So marketing in itself—usually not a subject taught in medical school or residency—becomes another reason for physicians to look to larger physician organizations that do those things necessary so the physician can concentrate on practicing medicine.

FIGURE 2–1

Evolution from Solo Practice to Group Practice

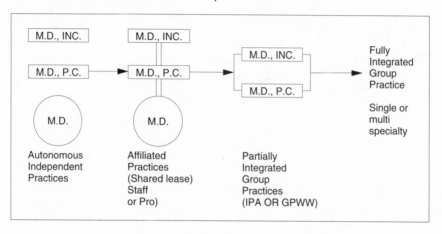

SUCCESS THROUGH CHANGE

The essence of change has obviously been different for physicians in different locations and in different specialties. *The end result, however, has been that physicians need to think about a way to think about change.* Obviously different physicians think about change in different ways depending on where their practices are; what type of practice they have; and their own personal, financial, and professional goals, as well as their age. To put the potential changes into perspective, I have included a series of charts basically showing the evolution from autonomous, independent practices, through to the formation of single specialty or multispecialty groups that might be considered fully integrated group practices. (See Figure 2–1.)

Figure 2–2 graphically displays how the clinic without walls, or the group practice without walls concept, might look in a given medical service area. This chart shows how the payors would contract with a group practice without walls having the authority to legally sign contracts. Such contracts would obligate physicians in their current practice locations to accept and treat certain patients potentially at a predetermined reimbursement level. This practice concept (group practice without walls or GPWW) was started in the middle 1980s. The concept is one

FIGURE 2-2

Group Practice without Walls

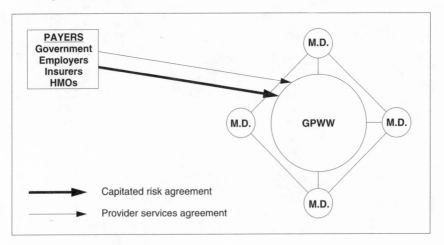

where a new professional entity is legally created through which revenues and expenses flow to contracted physicians and/or medical groups. There are economies of scale with this concept; often a central business unit can handle the administrative paperwork or those patients that are seen by the contracted physicians or medical groups under the contractual plans arranged and signed for by the group practice without walls leadership. The governance of such a group practice without walls usually includes representation from each of the practices participating in the GPWW. As with all types of physician organizations, the legal ramifications of this type of physician organization definitely need to be clarified up front before physicians can be obligated by the board or management of the group practice without walls. Regardless of the type of model that physicians may move into the future, they need to rely on competent and experienced health care legal and financial advisors to assist them in the transitions to one of the new organizations.

The next organizational model in Figure 2–3 is the MSO (management services organization or medical services organization). The MSO concept has a number of different hybrid models. However, for the purposes of this chapter I briefly point out a common underlying principle of most MSOs is that these are for-

FIGURE 2-3

Management Services Organization

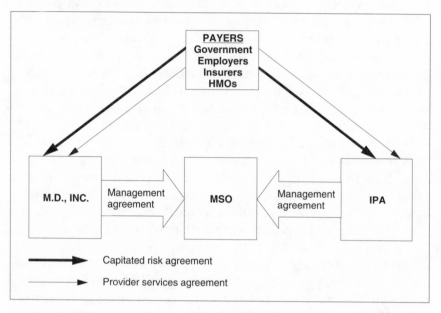

profit organizations and as such are taxable entities. The MSOs of today are owned by one or more entities; that is, hospitals, physicians, or investors. The activity of the MSO centers around the administration, management information system, support services, and often managed care contract negotiations the MSO provides on a contract basis to physicians, usually in medical groups. The physicians usually maintain ownership of their medical records and often control their medical practice patterns and income distribution; at the same time, they have purchased or contracted with the MSO to be responsible for the tangible assets of the medical group, its financial activities, and often the group's employees who usually are not actual health care providers.

THE GROWTH OF GROUP PRACTICES

Depending on the provider's location in the country, there has been a growing interest in developing or joining group practices by physicians coming out of residency, as well as by physicians who want to gain the benefits of membership and managed care participation through a larger organization. For example, the Medical Group Management Association in Denver, Colorado, now has several thousand medical groups as members in its organization. The American Group Practice Association in Alexandria, Virginia, is another national organization that has been responsive to medical groups' needs on a national level. Both organizations have in recent years worked closely with the American Medical Association, particularly on physician reimbursement issues and Medicare, as well as on insurance reform and health care reform activities.

There are estimated to be more than 20,000 group practices in the United States, depending on your definition of a group practice. Basically, a fairly standard definition of a group practice would be three or more physicians who have a common billing system and who have a common medical record for their patients and who are joined together organizationally. Obviously at the opposite end of the scale from this definition are the very large, multispecialty group practices such as the Mayo Clinic, the Cleveland Clinic, the Palo Alto Clinic, and the Lahey Clinic. Actually, many clinics in the country now have well over 50 physicians on their staff. Many of these medical groups have grown over the years to where they provide health care to patients in many, multiple locations. As an example, the Fargo Clinic of Fargo, North Dakota, has grown considerably over the last 15 years; now it has practice locations in more than 20 different sites. The Mayo Clinic which for years and years had strongly resisted requests to expand elsewhere, now has started two of its own large satellites in Jacksonville, Florida, and Scottsdale, Arizona, both approaching 100 physicians. At the same time, in the geographical area around Rochester, Minnesota, the Mayo Clinic has been aggressively acquiring physician practices. This acquisition mode over the last five years has resulted in Mayo Clinic Rochester now having 47 practice sites in Minnesota, northern Iowa, and western Wisconsin. Clearly the trend of the future is more and more physicians joining more and more group practices.

Often times, physicians and medical groups lacking capital reserves have turned to hospitals as a source of revenues for expansion or capitalization. A current model of this type of activity is called a PHO (physician-hospital organization). Figure 2–4 indicates that

FIGURE 2–4

Physician Hospital Organization (PHO)

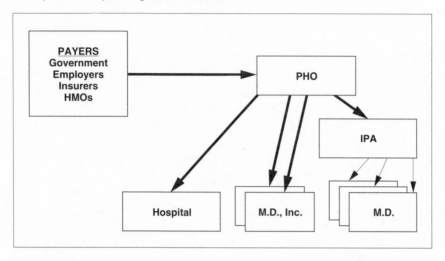

various third party-payors contract with the physician hospital organization that has subcontracted with a number of organizations but usually at least with a hospital and a medical group. While the new organization may be owned jointly by the hospital and a medical group/affiliated physicians, the entities themselves may maintain their independent status, and even potentially their same IRS tax status; that is, the hospital might be tax-exempt, whereas the physician organization may be taxable. Some PHOs may offer practice management services and/or might acquire the assets of a medical group. PHOs sometimes may be classified as having an opened or closed panel relationship for physicians who are not part of the governance of the PHO. Again various legal considerations need to be addressed, particularly at the governance level for newly developed PHOs. Once these are legally satisfied, however, the new organization can usually contract with third-party payers on a risk basis for both physician services and inpatient care.

The group practice of medicine can take many different avenues, potentially starting with a 3-physician single specialty practice up to the 1,000+ physicians in integrated multispecialty group practices such as the Mayo Clinic. Although the Mayo Clinic became a nonprofit foundation in 1914 when it turned over all of its assets to a foundation and all of its physicians went on salary, only in the last 10 to 20 years have some of the other very large integrated medical groups moved toward the medical foundation model. (See Figure 2–5.)

The medical foundation model has a number of variations throughout the country. The underlying principle linking foundation models is that they are usually nonprofit organizations from the standpoint of the Internal Revenue Service (IRS). Today, providers wishing to become medical foundations go through a rather lengthy legal process and, if approved, usually become classified by the IRS as a 501(c)(3) organization. Then, these organizations no longer have to pay taxes on any profit and as such have the opportunity to build up cash reserves.

Most physician organizations today are professional corporations that are taxable. Therefore, most professional medical corporations make a decision to distribute any revenues over expenses that exist on December 31 of each year so that those revenues will not be taxed from a corporate standpoint. Certainly from a short-term standpoint that is usually beneficial to the partners of the professional corporation. However, in the long run, the medical group does not have cash reserves when it needs to expand its physical facilities or invest in a new management information system. Therefore, the nonprofit foundation that does not pay taxes has the ability to create cash reserves and use those reserves for expansion of either physical facilities or acquiring medical practices or new medical equipment or larger management information systems.

THE MOVE TO INTEGRATED SYSTEMS AND RELATIONSHIPS

Figure 2–5 shows a nonprofit foundation that has developed a capitated risk agreement as well as an ownership/service agreement with a hospital. Although it would not be imperative for a large medical group to own a hospital before becoming a medical foundation (the Mayo Clinic operated for more than 50 years without owning a hospital) there are three main advantages to either ownership or having some type of legal relationship with a hospital. The first advantage would be that in many cases, a hospital appropriate to become a part of a foundation would already

FIGURE 2–5

Foundation Model

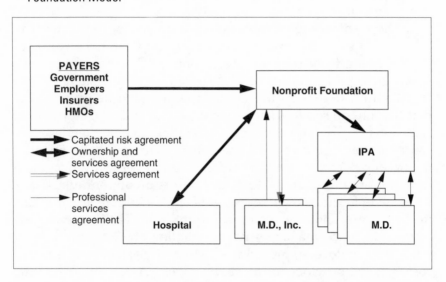

have a nonprofit status with the Internal Revenue Service. This could be used as a basis to build on for the physician organization to transition from a professional corporation into a medical foundation. A second major advantage for having a relationship with one or more hospitals is that under managed care the managed care company wants to shift as much financial risk as possible to the providers. When a hospital and medical group are part of the same medical foundation, they can negotiate contracts jointly to the combined benefit of the foundation, as opposed to individually negotiating contracts with a managed care organization benefiting one but not both of the provider organizations. The third advantage of the medical foundation model is that the foundation might have physicians as part of its own integrated group practice but that some specialty care (i.e., cardiac surgery) may not be represented on their staff. Therefore, they can contract directly with a specialist or group of specialists to provide the types of care they are currently not providing themselves so that in the managed care environment they can still represent all of the services that the managed care company wants to contract for and market to employers. As previously mentioned, the changes required for this type of entity, particularly to maintain the foundation's non-profit status, need to be approached very carefully, with very competent and experienced legal advice.

The medical foundation model has many of the benefits of what might be considered the end of the spectrum for physicians; that is, going from the solo practitioner to the other end of the spectrum as part of a vertically integrated delivery system.

Figure 2–6 depicts the vertically integrated delivery model that contains all services necessary to provide a total continuum of care. This is very important today in competitive marketplaces because the managed care companies often prefer to shift all financial risk to one contracting organization. Such a vertically integrated delivery organization system then needs a common electronic database to facilitate the integration of clinical, pharmacy, financial, managed care, and other contract information. The integrated services and unified management should allow the integrated delivery system to develop procedures so that the system can become a cost effective provider for all service lines. As we discuss in the next chapter, the various stages of managed care and the vertically integrated delivery system usually would not appear until stage four in managed care development in a given marketplace. Stage five might be represented by the vertically integrated system that has now gone beyond contracting with managed care companies to provide the total continuum of care. They will have developed their own managed care products to compete in the marketplace with traditional managed care companies. Such a possibility also potentially exists from the opposite approach of managed care companies acquiring enough hospitals and physician groups to become not only a managed care company but also a vertically integrated delivery system.

As I indicated earlier in this chapter, physicians need to think about ways to think about change. Obviously with the models described in this chapter, one of the key questions is who is the boss? In the new model organizations, will there be an authoritarian, autocratic approach to decision making? Under what circumstances would the physicians' best interests and the care of the physicians' patients be best met? It is assumed that the democratic process, whereby the majority rules, is a time-honored tradition in this country and often used by physician partnership. However, with

FIGURE 2-6

Health Care Delivery Vertical Integration Model

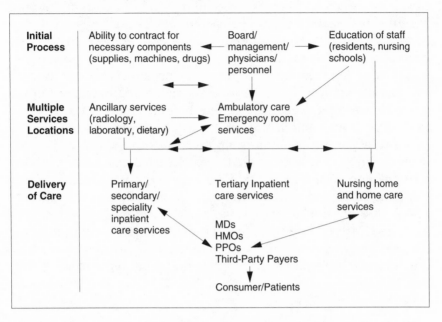

large organizations, particularly those that might be approaching $100 million a year or more, such a focus and management style may not be most appropriate. In certain of the models discussed, various state and federal regulations might require a specific type of decision-making process that often is representative, allowing for a hierarchical approach. This can be efficient; however, it also can be politically driven. Unfortunately for most physicians used to making their own decisions or having significant input into the decision-making process, their influence is now delegated to full-time professional executives. In some organizations, however, such executives are physicians.

As physicians move from one form of organization structure to the next to be more competitive in the managed care world, it is extremely important that there be broad constituent input into the planning process, to be followed by clear and consistent direction, with operational delegation and regular communication to providers, regardless of the model to be achieved. Because we are focusing on physicians' organizations providing patient care, it still remains very important that physicians receive adequate and timely information. They also should have adequate input into the approval of bylaws and/or changes in articles and bylaws. It has been my experience for successful ongoing operations that physicians need to have adequate input into incentives and income distribution systems, so that the physician's professional services are compensated in a truly appropriate manner recognizing the differences between managed care penetration and reimbursement in a given service area and its impact on physician compensation.

All of the previous information relates to the rapid changes in the format of how physicians practice medicine today. These changes and different models are primarily a reflection of the changing managed care environment in the physician's marketplace. As mentioned earlier, we discuss the multiple stages of managed care development in the next chapter. Similarly, we discuss the various models of managed care organizations as they transition from one stage of development to the next.

3

CHAPTER

The Stages of Managed Care Development and Their Impact on Physicians

Oliver Wendell Holmes wrote, "I find the great thing in this world is not so much where we stand as in what direction we are moving." Personally, as it relates to managed care, I would add to that quote "and how fast we are moving." The direction that managed care is moving and the pace of its change are the key factors behind the various types of physician organizations as responses to managed care development.

SHIFTING FINANCIAL RISK

As indicated in Chapter 1, managed care is here to stay and it has brought about continual changes. *Of key importance to providers today is that managed care often shifts the financial risk from the third-party payers and insurers to the providers.* Often times this is done with the hope by providers of an increase in the volume of patients they care for, or at least, the opportunity to maintain their patient market share in a given service area. Other changes impacting providers at the various stages of development of managed care will be an increased volume of discounts, as well as an increase in accountability and a focus on patient education and wellness.

FIGURE 3–1

Risks and Rewards of Provider Contracting

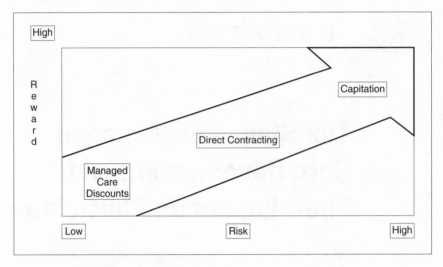

The diagram on the risks and rewards of provider contract-ing in Figure 3–1 put into perspective the wide range of models that managed care companies and plans have developed. We discuss this in the rest of this chapter.

Recognizing that most managed care companies and insur-ance companies with managed care products are in business to make a profit (even in Minnesota where HMOs are by law non-profit) the changes brought about by managed care organizations and their contracting are designed to increase their bottom line. A recent example of such change, which affects providers in more than 25 states, was the announcement in July 1995 that United Healthcare and MetraHealth were merging. The new organization has more than 8 million Americans receiving care from one of their many managed care plans in over 25 states. Their annual revenues from all services provided will be close to $6 billion a year.[1] However, it would be safe to assume that these figures are only a starting point for this new combined organization. In the middle 1980s, I worked for United Healthcare (UH) developing

---

[1]These figures appeared on p. 1, Section B in the *Minneapolis Star Tribune* on July 3, 1995.

new HMOs in different states across the country. I can assure you that the approach to contracting and dealing with physicians then was very different from what it is today and what it is likely to be in the future. With this new merger, United Healthcare can expand even further into more states and more metropolitan areas within states where the firm already has plans. This gives them much better access to national contracts, as well as much more leverage with local providers.

The purpose in describing the changes with United Healthcare is that this company is representative of what is happening with many of the managed care companies throughout the United States. The result is that the physicians who do contracting with United Healthcare, or other managed care organizations, must not assume that because they have signed a UH contract that their lives will now return to normal. In fact, even in the most mature managed care marketplaces today, such as Minneapolis/St. Paul, the changes in contracting and managed care are continuing and are likely to continue for years to come.

FIVE STAGES OF MANAGED CARE EVOLUTION

The changes at UH provide a good background to discuss the various stages of the managed care market evolution and form a backdrop for the various models of managed care that physicians and their administrators will be contracting with for years to come. *Realize that today the pace of managed care change, competition, and penetration is increasing rapidly.* Therefore, providers are moving faster through and from one stage of managed care market evolution to another.

Stage One

Recognizing that there are going to be differences within each stage and within each marketplace, a broad description of stage one would be a market such as Birmingham, Alabama, or Syracuse, New York. In this stage and, in similar markets today, there is little managed care, little hospital consolidation, and few large physician groups. There is likely to be an overuse of hospital inpatient care in relation to national standards.

Stage Two

In markets such as Atlanta, Orlando, or New York City, we find growing managed care that is mostly on a discounted fee-for-service basis, with some capitation starting. Also starting is some hospital consolidation in this type of marketplace. Becoming more of a trend in this stage are primary care physicians who are moving toward larger groups and physicians, in total, changing how they are organized. Also in many of the stage two and stage three markets, the hospitals have started to give deep price discounts in their contract negotiations because of the oversupply of beds.

Stage Three

The rate of change of health care providers in stage three becomes very much like a snowball gathering speed as it rolls down the mountainside. Not only does it gather speed but it also increases in size and sometimes produces an avalanche. In stage-three markets such as Detroit, Boston, Phoenix, and San Francisco, we now see heavy managed care penetration including some Medicare and Medicaid managed care programs. Today at least seven managed care organizations compete for the Medicaid business in the Phoenix market area.

Capitation, particularly for primary care physicians in stage three, has become a more routine part of managed care contract negotiations. There is an acceleration of primary care physicians to move to larger medical groups. Specialty physicians are organizing in a variety of different models to negotiate managed care contracts. Part of this acceleration is that managed care plans are becoming much more competitive and often start to drop physicians and hospitals from their plans, if the providers are not cost effective. At the end of the spectrum of stage three, there is a start in some markets for providers to develop continuums of care as providers and insurers begin to align.

Stage Four

Markets such as San Diego and Minneapolis that have more than 50 percent HMO penetration are categorized as stage four. In these cities, managed care reimbursement dominates provider payment arrangements, as there is very little fee-for-service left. Wherever providers and insurers become strongly aligned, they produce a few large health care systems that dominate the marketplace. Currently San Diego has two to three such systems and Minneapolis has three to four such systems depending on how you classify a system. These changes often produce a shift in physician supply, a dramatic reduction in the amount of fees to and services provided by specialists. Also physicians are moving toward larger and better organized physician/medical groups and other organizational models like MSOs and foundations. Although it is a potential factor in stage two and stage three, in stage four the purchasing of health care and contracting by employer coalitions can have a significant impact, similar to managed care, on providers. Services under such direct contracting arrangements reimburse providers a set fee while the providers are at financial risk for total services needed by the employees and their dependents.[2]

Stage Five

Stage five has been described as the end game. The end game is one where networks with significant market share form true partnerships with insurers. Another description of stage five might be one where integrated systems manage significant patient populations. Thus, no markets currently meet that description of stage five.

Quite frankly, I believe these descriptions of stage five are more likely to be at the end of stage four. I see stage five not necessarily as the end game but rather the future is now.[3] I

---

[2]The various stages just described were summarized from "How Markets Evolve." *Hospital and Health Networks,* APM, Inc., March 5, 1995, p. 48.

[3]John F. McCally and Roger Nauert, "Direct Contracting: The Future Is Now," *MGM Journal,* April 1993, pp. 23–24, 26, 28–29.

believe that stage five will be achieved when many employers with more than 250 employees and their employees jointly share the responsibility for both improved health and reducing the cost of their health care through coordinated and win-win contracted relationships with providers. Once the providers reach the end of stage four, they already are highly integrated, working toward improved cost efficiency, and usually involved with strong contractual relationships for providing health care services that focus on outcomes, quality, and cost effectiveness. How physicians become that integrated is the subject of the next chapter.

4

CHAPTER

Models for Physician Responses and Managed Care Participants

This book has been written for physicians and their financial and administrative advisors who are in the first three stages of managed care market evolution described in Chapter Three. However, it is also useful for physicians leaving residency or moving from a small practice to a larger practice or moving to a larger marketplace, where managed care has a much stronger penetration. For all those readers then, I list the backgrounds and diagrams for the various managed care models physicians can participate in or contract with or both.

STAFF MODEL HMO

Going back 50 years or more, particularly in California, we have seen the Kaiser model grow over the years. Kaiser now provides health care to millions of Americans not only in California but also on the East Coast and in other parts of the country. Basically, Kaiser uses the staff model HMO. In this type of HMO, the physician is actually employed by Kaiser. The administrative structure of Kaiser is designed to coordinate the health care services provided to the

FIGURE 4-1

Staff Model HMO

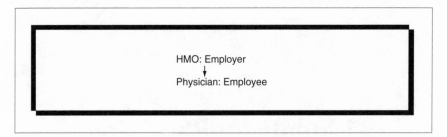

HMO provides health care services at its own facility, primarily through employed physicians.

FIGURE 4-2

Group Model HMO

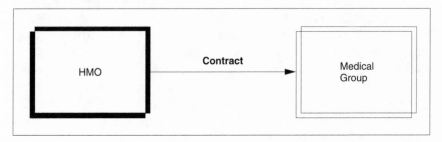

HMO provides health care services primarily through a single multispecialty medical group.

patient, usually by a primary care (gatekeeper) physician; it includes acute inpatient care and home health care. Kaiser and similar staff model HMOs also do the contracting with employers and with other providers as necessary, outside of those providers that are part of their own system. (See Figure 4–1.)

The staff model HMO is somewhat different depending on the organization and the members on the decision-making board. As an example, the board members of Group Health, Inc., of Minneapolis/St. Paul are elected representatives from its enrollees in the health plan. Group Health has been successful over the years in growing to more than 500,000 enrollees and its own hospital and

FIGURE 4-3

Network Model HMO

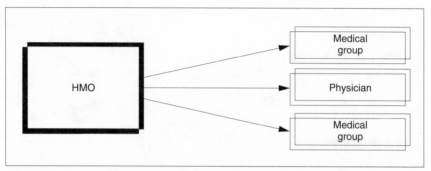

HMO provides health care services through contracts with individual physicians and medical groups.

now has merged with another managed care organization to provide services to a large business coalition and its employees at a fixed price. However, even though Group Health has the commonality of its staff model position, like Kaiser, with its physicians being employed, it also contracts with other physicians and medical groups in the community, so those providers are part of the Group Health Network, now called Health Partners.

GROUP MODEL HMO

The Group Model HMO is a managed care organization that contracts with, as opposed to employs, physicians primarily through a single multispecialty medical group. Depending on the size of the group and on its location, this is a somewhat self-limiting model unless the group practice has many multiple locations.

NETWORK MODEL HMO

Group models sometimes make a transition to become network model HMOs. In this situation, the HMO provides health care services through contracts with multiple physicians and medical groups. Often times the network model covers a large geographical area. However, because of the differences in contracting and

FIGURE 4-4

IPA Model HMO

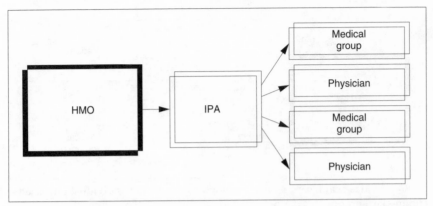

HMO provides health care services through contracts with an individual practice association, formed by or on behalf of physicians and medical groups. The IPA may be owned by or composed of gatekeepers/specialists.

with the integration of different groups that are contracted with, the outcomes and cost efficiency of this model are not necessarily uniform. (See Figure 4–3.)

INDEPENDENT PRACTICE OR PHYSICIAN ASSOCIATION (IPA) MODEL HMO

The IPA model HMO has significant appeal to a large group of physicians, often specialists, who may be signing up with more than one managed care organization. The concept for the IPA model is that a separate legal entity uses contracting as a mechanism for having adequate physicians and various services covered. The IPA becomes the administrative and financial focal point for contracting with the providers/managed care organization/employers. In such a model, the physicians as providers basically remain independent of each other with the potential for required protocols and referral mechanisms between the various providers of the IPA. (See Figure 4–4.)

FIGURE 4–5

Preferred Provider Organization Model

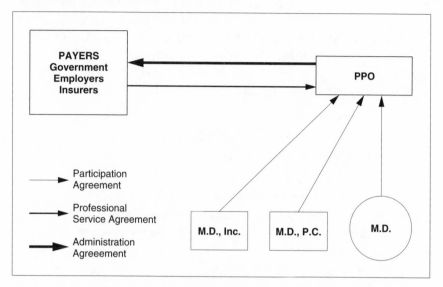

PREFERRED PROVIDER ORGANIZATION (PPO) MODEL

The PPO concept is very similar to the IPA concept. That is, a preferred provider organization is a new legal entity formed to negotiate contracts with third-party payors. Usually this allows the participating providers to retain their independence and autonomy. By and large, PPOs usually are open panel arrangements with discounted fee-for-service contracts. In these cases, the patients often use participating providers due to their lower professional fees/deductibles/copayments. (See Figure 4–5.) As physicians are confronted with new managed care contracts, particularly capitated contracts, everyone affected by the signing of those new contracts must be aware of who the contracting managed care company is and what its goal is in contracting with each physician or medical group. The preceding models of various HMOs and PPOs are basically just that—models; models can have many different approaches and designs. Remember there are already more than 1,000

HMOs and PPOs in the United States, all of which have different organizational arrangements with providers and approaches to achieving the same goal (i.e., to make money for the organization). The managers of these HMOs and PPOs are often rewarded at the end of the year on how well they do in achieving profitability. Therefore, as physicians and their administrators start to negotiate contracts with managed care organizations, they must research:

Who the company is.

What are its goals and objectives.

Who are their key employees.

What is their experience.

What are their personal goals.

What is the relationship administratively between the negotiation team and management of the managed care organization.

Who are the real decision makers.

In doing research on managed care organizations, as well as when analyzing managed care contracts, it is vital to understand the terminology used in the industry. Therefore, we have included a glossary of managed care contract, managed care capitation, and actuarial terminology. There have been horror stories of physicians and medical groups who signed managed care contracts because they thought the contract rate was OK but neglected to read, understand, or analyze the rest of the contract. When I was a national consultant for a Big Six accounting and consulting firm, I assisted a client that had lost millions of dollars due to a major contract that was signed because they thought the price was right and didn't recognize the financial risk impact of the other clauses in the contract. I want to emphasize that it is vital to understand the impact of the entire contract, and not just the reimbursement. Recognizing that the contract terminology in the glossary is boring, I still recommend that it not only be read but also understood and certainly referred to in the process of contract analysis and negotiation.

5

CHAPTER

Major Contract Issues That Impact Physicians in Managed Care Contracts

As mentioned earlier, with more than 1,000 managed care companies having multiple managed care plans, thousands of managed care contracts are now in effect between managed care organizations and physicians/other providers. Many of those contracts are tailor-made to the specifications of the employer, particularly for self-insured employers. Additionally, as many specialty physicians already realize, there can be a series of subcontracts between a PHO, an MSO, or a medical group that wants to subcontract with other providers for some of the services and risk that they have assumed under a singular, total contract with a managed care company or employer. Given all these variables, this chapter focuses on the various contract issues that have a major impact on physicians practices, in addition to the actual reimbursement rate. In several of the following chapters, we also discuss how to analyze and determine the appropriateness of the reimbursement rate for the contracts with specific physicians/medical group practices.

Whenever analyzing a contract proposed by a managed care company, keep in mind that this contract was prepared by its legal and management departments to benefit the managed care company. And, unless the managed care company is just starting out, assume that many of the clauses in this contract have been developed because in previous contracts with providers situations arose that the managed care organization is trying to eliminate in the future. Some of these clauses benefit both the managed care company and the providers. More often, the majority of the clauses and these contracts are proposed for the protection and the benefit (profit) of the managed care company.

In certain states, managed care contracts need to have the approval of the state department of insurance or the state department of health. Simply because the contracts have received such approval from a state agency does not mean that such contracts protect providers during a disagreement down the road. Usually, the state regulatory agency bases its approval of contracts on what it considers appropriate for the patients receiving care under those contracts. Whether a contract is biased toward the managed care organization and allows that MCO to be more profitable is irrelevant to the regulatory agency's disapproval or approval of the contract.

Many physicians and their business managers or administrators approach the typical 20 to 40 pages of a managed care contract with some fear and trepidation. Usually this is caused by their lack of understanding of how contracts are structured and how those various clauses, if accepted, impact their specific practice of medicine, both operationally and financially. Later in this book, I emphasize that providers can maintain or increase their financial viability through managed care and capitated contracts. At the same time, I include the caveat that it is not just the reimbursement rate that is important, depending on what is included in the contract and how those clauses are negotiated multiple aspects of the contract financially impact providers. Typically, the following are key parts of a managed care contract:

◆ The contract type and parties to the contract.
◆ The specifics and listing of what services are covered in a contract for a reimbursement to be paid to the provider.
◆ Clarification of how and who determines the medical necessity for providing those services to be covered as included in the previous point.
◆ Definitions of where and when those services in the previous two points will be provided, specifically to include emergency care definitions.

◆ Reimbursement mechanism/timing for the provision of approved services.

◆ Risk-sharing arrangements/outlier clauses.

◆ Specifics of the reconciliation process and timing of any payments.

◆ Volume/length of stay/other incentives.

◆ Review/access/ownership of medical records.

◆ Access to/data required by managed care organizations from providers.

◆ Hold harmless clauses.

◆ Grievance/dispute procedures.

◆ Legalese relating to a variety of issues such as how notices are to be given and which state law governs the contract.

Because most contracts are likely to be different, even though you understand a similar clause in another contract, analyze each of the key contract clauses in the current contract. By doing so you can become aware of the impact each clause will have on your practice. As an example, in the first key clause just mentioned, you should understand who is the contracting organization and what is their financial stability. Over the last 10 years, numerous HMOs and PPOs have either gone out of business, gone into bankruptcy, merged with another company, or been acquired by another organization. In some instances, the MCO or insurance company may have a national reputation but be new to your particular service area. In these circumstances, you want to determine the likelihood of the MCO being successful in your service area. As was pointed out, this particular clause at the front of the contract defines who the MCO is and who the provider is (usually a specific physician, medical group, MSO, hospital or PHO). However, the success of the plan and your participation in it may very strongly be aligned with which other providers are contracted by the managed care organization. Therefore, in this section you must determine the other providers who are or may become members of the MCO's panel or who are also accepting financial risk with the same MCO.

Also important is the part of the contract that specifies what services the provider is expected to provide for a given reimbursement. Many times the contract calls for an attachment or addendum to the contract to specify specific services. Again, there will be times when this information actually is not attached to the contract physicians are asked to review and sign. Not only should physicians and their administrators have the opportunity to review all covered services before signing the contract but they also should negotiate as part of the contract the opportunity to approve the addition of any new services, or if not approving the service, to at least approve the reimbursement for such services added to the contract.

Often times when reviewing a contract's covered services, physicians assume that their judgment of when such services should be provided would not be questioned. In reality, many contracts include a clause that stipulates that the covered services, "when medically necessary," are reimbursed to the provider who gives those services to the patient. The key here is to have in writing a definition of what the managed care organization considers medically necessary. Sometimes physicians feel comfortable having the MCO medical director make such a decision. Often times the definition of a medical necessity or standards of good medical practice can be interpreted in different ways by different individuals. Certainly, if possible, the definitions should reflect the physician's medical judgment based on the medical condition of a given patient. If the MCO's medical director or a triage nurse makes the decision, providers should try to negotiate the opportunity to provide input into the hiring and firing of medical directors.

The whole issue of what services are covered based on the patient's condition at the time of service brings up a very related issue often overlooked or not well defined in contracts and one that is potentially very expensive. That is a clause defining a medical emergency, who authorizes such care, and most important to the provider who provides the care, who pays for that care if the patient goes into the emergency room on the weekend and is not seen by the physician/provider group signing his contract. Of similar concern, and often a clause to be clarified, is that concerning when physicians tell patients over the phone that they should go to the emergency room but where the managed care contract with the patients indicates that emergency room treatment is only authorized and reimbursable when the patient has gone through a nurse triage process, usually via the phone.

A number of individual items under reimbursement are very important, such as the specific rate of reimbursement, that is, a capitated rate of specific dollars per member per month (PMPM), or a percentage of the premium, or a specific discount from usual and customary. If it is a discount from the usual and customary, an important point of clarification is whose definition of usual and customary is used and at what time (i.e., the time of signing the contract, or the preceding year, or as usual and customary at certain specified dates during the lifetime of the contract).

Particularly under capitation, the contract should spell out in great detail what are the risk sharing arrangements, if any. As already stated, the focus under capitation is often for the managed care organization to shift as much of the financial risk as possible to the providers. Assuming the physician/medical groups are organized to accept financial risk, the contracts must spell out at what point the risk sharing arrangement takes effect and who is tracking whether or not the risk sharing arrangement is actually being implemented. As an example, if the providers accept the financial risk for the first $10,000 for any given patient under capitation, and if a certain patient has $12,000 worth of care, who is going to indicate that the $10,000 risk sharing arrangement limit has been reached, who will pay for the services over and above $10,000, and when will that payment be made.

Speaking of tracking the expenses under capitation, another very key aspect that needs to be clarified in the contract is the tracking, reporting, and reconciliation of incurred but not recorded (IBNR) claims. During the course of most managed care capitated contracts, particularly with primary care physicians but also with some specialists, certain patients are referred for care to specialists or hospitals not under the same risk contract. When those noncapitated providers finish providing care to the original doctor's patients, they are going to send their bills to either the managed care organization or the referring provider. Not only should the referral process of the patient be clarified in the contract but also what happens to the bill from the provider outside of the contract and at what point will those expenses be charged back to the referring capitated provider. The expenses of patients referred out of the capitated plan arrangement are considered IBNR. As we discuss in a later chapter, accounting for IBNR becomes very important to ensure financial stability and success. When the contract calls for the provider to track IBNR expense and pay approved IBNR claims, often times the providers must either upgrade or buy a new computer or new software to stay on top of this vital area.

Utilization review and quality assurance clauses (UR/QA) often provide a statement relating to the ownership and control of patient medical records. The MCO may want to claim ownership to the patient records or have as part of the contract the ability to review all patient records. This may or may not be a particular problem for the provider/medical group signing the contract. However, if the MCO is going to request multiple records be duplicated and sent to them for review, the contract should spell out who will pay for the duplication and mailing cost, as well as the time frame the providers have to respond to the MCO's request.

The issue of nonmedical information gathering and reporting is equally important. Obviously there is a cost to developing and providing information to a managed care company. A potential confidentiality issue also can be involved, depending on what data the managed care company is requiring to be sent to them. In the contractual language, a rather innocuous clause may be included: "the provider will be required to report certain financial information relating to the care of patients." Such a clause could mean that the MCO will request on its own form information related to the services provided, and the reimbursement received for those services for all of the patients cared for by the provider. This means that you and your staff will have to pull together the information and present it to them in the way that they want it. This would be not only time consuming but also potentially provide the managed care organization (and others who may have access to that information) with information that could be detrimental to the providers, particularly when they are renegotiating the contract in the future.

Speaking of renegotiating the contract, usually toward the end of the managed care contract one or two clauses relate to the term of the contract and the termination of the contract. Both of these areas are certainly very important. If the contract has a one-year renewable term, the MCO must clarify if the term is automatically renewed when neither side provides notice to the other side to the contrary and if so at what contract rate will it be renewed.

At the same time, if the managed care organization or the provider wishes to terminate the contract, the time frame for such a termination needs to be spelled out. And, of equal importance, is what happens to the patients under care during both the time of the notice of termination and after the contract has terminated. During this time both the provider and the provider's patients should know who is going to pay for the care being provided and when that care should be paid for.

Toward the end of the contract, there are a series of what might be called legalese clauses. Although seemingly not harmful, physicians and medical groups should have competent managed care advisors and attorneys assisting them with the contract analysis and negotiation activity. Nowhere is this more important than toward the end of the contract where there are various issues such as hold harmless clauses, dispute resolution, and assignment of contracts. Although most providers do not spend much time thinking about either the managed care organization or the provider going into bankruptcy, such events do occur today. I strongly recommend that physicians in medical groups have any contract clause relating to potential bankruptcy, as well as any applicable governing state laws, reviewed by competent legal council.

Speaking of these legalese issues, usually at the end of the contract, you may want to ensure that the appeals process allows for you to defend yourself in the question of standards of care. At the same time providers may best get a clarification as to whether or not their malpractice company/attorney can represent them or whether another attorney might have to be retained in such cases. Because more and more health care is being delivered under the specifics of a managed care contract, the preceding discussion of various contract clauses and their potential impact raises the issue of when physicians should or should not sign a contract. Often this question can be answered best by going through the practice analysis described in the next chapter.

6
CHAPTER

Analyze Your Current Practice Activity before Looking at a Contract

As we discussed in the last chapter, many aspects of the managed care contract may significantly impact not only a physician's practice but also the bottom line of the financial statement. To truly understand the impact of various managed care contracts, however, each practice needs to analyze what is currently happening in the practice. Many physicians/groups simply take the approach that they need only to know how much is being grossed each year to decide how to cut costs to increase their net take home compensation. However, that is not sufficient information when you are entering contracts that intentionally reduce the amount of gross revenue being paid, potentially put the physician at financial risk for many patients' care, or eliminate the opportunity to provide services to a segment of the patient population if the contract is not signed by the provider/group.

Therefore, physicians must truly understand the current dynamics of a provider's practice. Once this is done providers can impact their bottom line. There are many ways to look at the practice and results of that practice. Many current medical software systems give the answers to some or all of the financial questions in the rest of this chapter. However, the analysis of the answers to these questions is important when making decisions about signing or not signing proposed managed care contracts. The following 19 questions and their answers can not only be beneficial for the physician and group management in making decisions about signing a particular contract but also provide a thorough understanding for future trending of the information. This information can assist providers in developing a total managed care strategy to use in approaching managed care contracts. Although the 19 questions are relatively straightforward, some may need to be changed to reflect a particular physician/medical group practice. Another possible change, particularly for group practices, may be to analyze the answers to these questions on a per physician or per specialty basis. Questions 15 through 19 may be eliminated if the practice currently does not have any managed care/capitated contracts. For those physicians and those group practices that have been fortunate enough to not have managed care contracts to date, the information gathered about their own practice through this practice activity analysis will assist in the development of a managed care strategic plan for the future.

PRACTICE ACTIVITY ANALYSIS

1. Total number of active patients:

   Current year   _____

   Previous year   _____

   Preceding year   _____

   Percent of active patients (current year) who are:

Total Age Distribution		Male	Female
Under 18	_____	_____	_____
18–35	_____	_____	_____
36–50	_____	_____	_____
51–64	_____	_____	_____
65+	_____	_____	_____
Total	_____	_____	_____

2. Average number of visits per active patient per year:

   Current year   _____

   Previous year   _____

   Preceding year   _____

   Average charge per patient visit:

   Current year   _____

   Previous year   _____

   Preceding year   _____

3. Average number of new patients (never seen before in practice) per year:

   Current year   _____

   Previous year   _____

   Preceding year   _____

4. Total referrals from the practice to specialists per year:

   Current year   _____

   Previous year   _____

   Preceding year   _____

   List the three categories of medical/surgical specialties to which you most frequently refer patients:

   _____

   _____

   _____

5. Total patients referred to the practice per year:

   Current year   _____

   Previous year   _____

   Preceding year   _____

List the three most prevalent sources of patient referrals to
the practice by specialty categories or other referral
sources (self-referrals, referred by other patients, ancillary
health care professionals, etc.)

_____

_____

_____

6. Average referral income per patient, per year:

Current year   _____

Previous year   _____

Preceding year   _____

7. Average number of in-office ancillary service units per
patient, per year (list each procedure for which you charge
separately):

		Year	
Procedure	**Current**	**Previous**	**Preceding**
Laboratory	_____	_____	_____
EKG	_____	_____	_____
X-ray	_____	_____	_____
Other main diagnostic procedures			
_____	_____	_____	_____
_____	_____	_____	_____
_____	_____	_____	_____
Treatment procedures			
_____	_____	_____	_____
_____	_____	_____	_____
Total practice revenue (including revenues for laboratory and X-ray services)_____	_____	_____	

	Year		
Procedure	Current	Previous	Preceding
Total expense (including physician compensation)	_____	_____	_____
Total office expenses, (i.e., supplies and so on)	_____	_____	_____
Total other expenses (including charges from ancillary vendors paid by the practice)	_____	_____	_____
Average annual expenses per patient visit (Divide sum of expenses by number of active patients. Divide this total by average number of patient visits to obtain	_____	_____	_____
Average Annual Expense per Patient Visit	_____	_____	_____

9. Percent of active patients by principal source of payment:

	Year		
Source of Payment	Current	Previous	Preceding
Commercial/FFS	_____	_____	_____
Medicare	_____	_____	_____
Medicaid	_____	_____	_____
Self-Pay	_____	_____	_____
HMOs/PPOs (list by name)			
_____	_____	_____	_____
_____	_____	_____	_____
_____	_____	_____	_____
_____	_____	_____	_____
_____	_____	_____	_____

10. Determine the average length of time for outstanding receivables for the payors identified in question 9.

| | Days | | | |
Payor	30	60	90	90+
Commercial/FFS	_____	_____	_____	_____
Medicare	_____	_____	_____	_____
Medicaid	_____	_____	_____	_____
Self-Pay	_____	_____	_____	_____
HMOs/PPOs	_____	_____	_____	_____

11. List the companies that employ a significant number of patients within the practice.

Employer	System Offered by Employer	Number of Patients	Percent of Active Patients
_____	_____	_____	_____
_____	_____	_____	_____
_____	_____	_____	_____

12. Average patients seen in office per week:

Current year   _____

Previous year   _____

Preceding year   _____

Estimated additional capacity

_____ patients per week

13. Average number of hopital patient visits or consults per week:

Current year   _____

Previous year   _____

Preceding year   _____

Average number of hospital procedures (diagnostic and surgical) performed per week:

Current year   _____

Previous year   _____

Preceding year   _____

Average charge for hospital visits:

Current year   _____

Previous year   _____

Preceding year   _____

14. Number of requests for patient record transfers by reason for request:

Reason for Transfer Request	Year		
	Current	Previous	Preceding
Patient moving out of area	_____	_____	_____
Patient enrolled in HMO(List)	_____	_____	_____
_____	_____	_____	_____
_____	_____	_____	_____
_____	_____	_____	_____
Other(list reasons given by patients)			
_____	_____	_____	_____
_____	_____	_____	_____
_____	_____	_____	_____
Totals	_____	_____	_____

Analysis of Impact of Potential Managed Care System Participation

15. List the standard services covered by the system that are not part of the routine office practice (e.g., annual physicals for all patients). This information may best be determined by reviewing the physician contract and a copy of an employee benefit handbook.

Name of the System   **Services Covered (not routine)**

_____   _____
_____   _____
_____   _____
_____   _____
_____   _____

16. Procedures and treatments common to the practice that are not reimbursed separately by the system or are included as part of the system capitation rate.

Name of the System   **Services Covered (not routine)**

_____   _____
_____   _____
_____   _____
_____   _____
_____   _____

17. Number and average charge of those procedures and treatments most frequently performed in the practice:

Procedure/ Treatment	Number Per- formed per Year	Average Charge/ Procedure/ Treaments	Average Annual Revenue/ Procedure/ Treatments	Potential System Reim- burse- ment	*Difference
_____	_____	_____	_____	_____	_____
_____	_____	_____	_____	_____	_____
_____	_____	_____	_____	_____	_____
_____	_____	_____	_____	_____	_____

*Difference between Average Annual Revenue/Procedure/ Treatment and Potential Annual System Reimbursement.

18. If system reimbursement is based on capitation rates, how do these rates compare to the estimated average annual patient expenses?

System	Capitation Rate ($/Patient/Year)	Average Annual Expense per Patient*
_____	_____	_____
_____	_____	_____
_____	_____	_____
_____	_____	_____
_____	_____	_____
_____	_____	_____

*Sum of Expense divided by Active Patients equals Average Annual Expense per Patient.

19. For those systems with a withhold (risk assumption) pool, how is the withhold structured?

System	Percent Withheld from Primary Care Physician	Percent Withheld from Specialists
_____	_____	_____
_____	_____	_____
_____	_____	_____

7 CHAPTER

Fifty Questions to Improve Your Bottom Line and Negotiation Strategy

Literally hundreds of questions may be raised during the process of analyzing and negotiating a managed care contract, particularly a capitated contract. Certainly the number of questions also depend on the amount of managed care capitation in your particular marketplace, the particular managed care organization, and the contract it is proposing. Some questions were already pointed out in Chapter 5 as key contract issues. The following 50 questions are a starting point for your analysis of any new contract presented to you. In the next chapter, you can apply the questions and comments from Chapters 5 and 6, as well as the following 50 questions to actual sample capitated contracts. Of particular interest for those physicians and medical groups treating Medicare patients is the sample Medicare contract in Chapter 8, which could be greatly improved from the provider's standpoint if many of these questions were asked and answered during the negotiation process.

The order of these 50 questions, again recognizing that there could be many more, basically follows the somewhat standard placement of key clauses in a typical contract as outlined in Chapter 5.

1. Has the MCO been registered/approved by the state insurance department?

2. Who are the members of the MCO's board of directors and how are they elected?

3. In the marketing material, are the board members' specialties listed (if doctors) and may they be used as references?

4. Has the representative for the MCO provided you a list of employer groups that would be eligible to use your services if you signed their contract?

5. In how many counties in the state and in how many states does the MCO have contracts to provide similar services?

6. Has the MCO agreed or offered to share with you the types of contracts used by the MCO with other providers in other counties or other states?

7. Does the MCO carry professional liability insurance that covers providers?

8. Does the MCO require providers to carry a specific amount of liability insurance that may be higher than the provider currently has in force with his or her malpractice insurance carrier?

9. Has the provider received written confirmation that the insurance products the MCO offers are valid and legally marketable?

10. Does the contract require utilization reviews/quality assurance-type activities and, if so, are any of them done on a contract basis for the MCO by an outside company or agency?

11. Does the MCO currently have under investigation any professional liability issues or disputes or any such litigation in the courts?

12. Does the MCO currently have or have they had over the last three years any investigations by either state or federal agencies?

13. Does the contract contain any blank spaces?

14. Does the contract spell out how the physician/medical group can terminate the contract?

15. Does the contract spell out how much advance notice is required for either party to terminate the contract?

16. Does the contract attempt to incorporate by reference into the contract various documents the physician has not reviewed, such as a utilization review plan?

17. Does the contract hold harmless and indemnify the MCO from any liability arising from the physicians rendering a professional service without a mutual hold harmless clause for the provider from the managed care organization?

18. Is the contract an exclusive contract, prohibiting the physician from contracting with other managed care organizations?

19. Does the contract restrict the physician's referral patterns by requiring that referrals be made only to contracting physicians in groups that have contracted with the MCO?

20. Does the contract allow for the contract to be unilaterally amended by the MCO without the agreement of the physician/medical group?

21. Do all of the clauses in the contract relating to physician/patient medical records and confidentiality comport with state law?

22. Does the contract require that each physician member of a professional corporation or partnership execute the contract agreement?

23. Does a contractual requirement that the physician submit to arbitration any contractual dispute and/or professional liability dispute affect the physician's existing professional liability insurance coverage?

24. What impact does the termination of the contract have on the physician/patient relationship?

25. Does the contract require the physician to keep proprietary information confidential and if so for how long?

26. Does the contract make nonspecific reference to cost effective and quality care services?

27. Has a representative of the MCO made any important oral or written representations/promises relating to the physicians' contractual relationship which is not in the written contract?

28. Does the contract limit the physician's professional judgment regarding the involvement of specific additional physicians such as an anesthesiologist or assistant surgeon?

29. Does the contract limit the time for the physician/medical group to accurately submit claims?

30. Does the contract provide for the payment of clean claims to the physician/medical group within a specified time limit?

31. Does the contract provide for an interest payment if actual payment to the physician/medical group for approved services is delayed?

32. Does the contract require that the physician verify patient eligibility prior to providing service?

33. Does the contract clearly define and specify noncovered services?

34. Does the contract provide that the patient is liable for payment of noncovered services or that the patient cannot be billed for such services?

35. Does the contract allow/imply/state the physician's/group name will be used on brochures, or in other advertising on radio or TV?

36. Does the contract list the specific procedures or services that require prior authorization from the MCO to receive reimbursement?

37. Does the contract require that the physician modify existing office procedures and/or billing systems and, if so, is there any compensation to be paid to the physician to cover that cost?

38. Does the contract obligate the physician to provide any services after the contract is terminated?

39. Does the contract allow for the fee schedule/reimbursement to be unilaterally changed by the MCO without prior notice or without the prior approval of the physician/medical group?

40. Does the contract require physicians to arrange with another contract physician for coverage during absences and vacations?

41. Does the contract refer to unspecified medical policies?

42. Does any party to the contract have the right to unilaterally change medical policies?

43. Does the contract provide an opportunity to examine the experience and qualifications of those physicians required to be used as referral physicians for certain patient services?

44. Does the contract limit the right of a physician to contract with any other third-party/managed care organization?

45. Does the contract specifically exclude from coverage certain services rendered by various specialties?

46. Does the contract provide for a gatekeeper approach to the delivery of patient services?

47. Does the contract contain broadly worded indemnification clauses that shift risk from the MCO to the physician/medical group?

48. Does the contract directly or indirectly interfere with the physician's exercise of sound medical judgment?

49. Does the managed care organization assume liability for payments to providers when care is provided to patients after the patients have terminated without the MCO notifying the provider?

50. Can the contract be renewed automatically without future discussions or contracts signed?

8
CHAPTER

Analysis and Review of Sample Capitated and Medicare Contracts

After reviewing and understanding Chapters 5 through 7, physicians and administrators should now be ready to take a look at two sample contracts that were acutally in force at the time of this writing. Reading the various clauses in these contracts should now create a fair number of questions, from those in Chapters 5 through 7 or from the contract's specific clauses.

Many questions can be raised about the clauses in these two contracts. That is not to say these are necessarily bad contracts. Keep in mind that typical contracts are put together by the administration and legal counsel of the managed care organizations for the benefit of the managed care organization. Hopefully, they are not at the detriment of the physicians/providers signing the contract. Because physicians/providers can improve their financial arrangements and situations by understanding, clarifying, and negotiating all issues of the contract—not just the reimbursement rate—we have spent a fair amount of effort in this book on the total contract. As you review the sample contracts in this chapter, you will get a much better idea of the relevance and importance of the individual contract clauses and why we raised the questions discussed in Chapters 5 through 7. Following the review of these two sample contracts are some specific questions that could logically be raised in doing an analysis of these two contracts.

SAMPLE CONTRACTS

SAMPLE

PHYSICIAN AGREEMENT

PHYSICIAN AGREEMENT dated as of this _____ day of _____, 19_____, between_____ of _____ (state), a_____ Corporation and _____, [M.D.], who is either a physician of medicine or _____ _____specialty), licensed to practice in the (county/commonwealth) of _____(state), or a professional corporation or partnership comprised of physicians licensed to practice medicine or _____(specialty) in the county/commonwealth) of _____(state). This Agreement will be effective [date] _____, 19_____.

RECITAL:

_____ operates a health maintenance organization in the Service Area (PLAN) described in the attached Appendix D which has undertaken to arrange for the provision of medical care to its Subscribers and their Dependents (such Subscribers and their eligible Dependents entitled to service from the Plan are hereinafter referred to as "Members.")

1.   DEFINITIONS

        1.1   Definitions. As used in this Agreement, the following terms shall have the meanings set forth below.
        1.1.1.   "Coordination of Benefits" (COB) means the procedures set forth in the Subscription Agreement to determine which coverage is primary for payment of benefits to Members with duplicate coverage.
        1.1.2.   "Dependent" means an individual who qualifies as a Dependent under the terms and conditions of the Subscription Agreement.
        1.1.3.   "Encounter Form" means the form provided to Physician by _____for the reporting of medical services delivered by the Physician.
        1.1.4.   "Hospital Services" means (i) services provided under the Subscription Agreement by an entity which is licensed, certified, and operates as a hospital, (ii) services for chemical dependency, (iii) Medical

Services outside the Plan Service Area, and (iv) any other Medical Services not specifically included as services covered by the Primary Physician Capitation or as Referral Services.

1.1.5.   "Medical Director" means that physician designated by _____ to perform the duties of Medical Director as set forth in this Agreement and in accordance with the policies of _____.

1.1.6.   "Medical Services" means all services furnished to a Member pursuant to the Subscription Agreement.

1.1.7.   "Member" means an eligible subscriber or Dependent as defined in the applicable Subscription Agreement.

1.1.8.   "Participating Physician" means a primary care physician practicing in the Service Area who has entered into a contract substantially similar to this Agreement and who is not employed by or otherwise affiliated with Physician.

1.1.9.   "Per Member Maximum" means the per Member – per year limitations on referral or hospital charges as established by _____, from time to time.

1.1.10.   "Physician" is defined in the Preamble to this Agreement.

1.1.11.   "Physician Office Network" shall mean a physician network, an individual practice association or a medical group which has entered into an agreement with _____ to provide health care services to _____ Members, has as its primary purpose the delivery or arrangement for the delivery of health care services, and has entered into written service or employment agreements or other arrangements with health care professionals, the majority of whom are licensed to practice medicine . . .

1.1.12.   "Plan" means the health maintenance organization operated by _____ in the Service Area

1.1.13.   "PMPM" means per-Member/per-Month.

1.1.14.   "Preferred Providers" means providers approved by and designated by _____ as Preferred Providers from time to time.

1.1.15.   "Primary Physician Capitation" means the amount paid to each Physician monthly for services based on the age, sex and number of the Members selecting Physician.

1.1.16.   "Referral Services" means Medical Services arranged for by Physician and provided outside Physician's office other than Hospital Services.

1.1.17.   "Service Area" means the area described in Appendix D.

1.1.18.   "Subrogation" means the recovery of the cost of services and benefits provided to Members by _____ for which other parties are liable.

sample – only

1.1.19.   "Subscriber" means the employee or individual with whom _____ enters into, or who is the direct beneficiary of, a Subscription Agreement.

1.1.20.   "Subscription Agreement" means both group and individual contracts between _____ an employer or individual pursuant to which _____ provides Medical and Hospital Services, as such agreement may be amended from time to time.

The parties agree as follows:

2.   RELATIONSHIP OF PARTIES

2.1.   Relationship of the Entities, _____ and Physician are independent entities, and neither party is the agent, employee or servant of the other.

3.   PHYSICIAN-PATIENT RELATIONSHIP

3.1   Agreement to Accept Members. At the time of enrollment, a member shall be entitled to select from the list of Participating Physicians, including Physician, that Participating Physician from which the member wishes to receive the "Medical Services" covered by the Subscription Agreement pertaining to the Member, subject to the ability of such physician to accept additional Members under the agreement between the physician and _____. If Physician is so selected by a Member to provide Medical Services, Physician shall not refuse to offer Medical Services to the Member provided the Member has been certified by _____ as being eligible and provided the minimum number of Members set forth in Appendix A or, if Physician is already treating more Members than the minimum set forth in appendix A, of refusing to accept additional Members provided Physician shall have given _____ ninety (90) days prior written notice of such refusal.

3.2.   Transfer of Members. Because the physician-patient relationship is a personal one and may become unacceptable to either party, Physician may request, in writing, to _____ that a Member be transferred to another Participating Physician. Physician shall not, however, seek to have a Member transferred because of the amount of Medical Services required by the Member or because of the physical condition of the Member. Physician acknowledges that Members have a contractual right with _____ to request to be transferred to another Participating Physician. All such transfers subsequently approved shall become effective as soon as administratively feasible, but in any event within sixty (60) days from the date of request.

sample – only

3.3.   Other _____ Products. Physician agrees to provide services to patients participating in other products of _____ or its affiliates on a discounted fee-for-service basis according to the rates and fees set forth in Appendix E.

4.   FINANCIAL CONSIDERATIONS

4.1.   Primary Physician Capitation

4.1.1.   Primary Physician Capitation. _____ shall make monthly payments to Physician based on the age, sex and number of Members enrolled in Physician's practice as specified in Appendix B. Payments shall be made to Physician no later than the tenth working day of the month.

4.1.2.   Services Covered by Primary Physician Capitation. The Primary Physician Capitation is payment for professional services available on a 24-hour per day basis, laboratory services, medical supplies dispensed from the Physician's office, injectables, preventive care, or other services provided by Physician's staff, covering physicians, or call partners at the office, hospital, skilled nursing facility, patient's home or any other location where primary care is provided. Examples of services covered by the Primary Physician Capitation are listed in Appendix C. In no case will Physician be required to pay for Referral Services from Primary Physician Capitation.

4.2   Medical Management Fund

4.2.1.   Medical Management Fund. _____ shall establish a Participating Physicians' Medical Management Fund ("Medical Management Fund"), to recognize the importance of efficiently managing the entire treatment process for _____ Members. Each month, _____ shall credit the Medical Management Fund in the amount of $0.50 for each Member. The PMPM amount to be credited to the Medical Management Fund may be adjusted from time to time at the discretion of _____.

4.2.2.   Eligibility for Distributions. If Physician meets the eligibility criteria established from time to time, Physician will participate in the distribution from the Medical Management Fund pursuant to Section 4.2.4   Only those Physician Practices serving at least 200 _____ Members are eligible to participate in the Medical Management Fund. In addition, eligibility to receive the maximum distributions shall be conditioned upon the Physician Practice remaining open to accept new Members during a specific period of the year.

4.2.3.   Cost Target. For purposes of evaluating the efficiency of Participating Physicians' treatment patterns, _____ shall, on a quarterly basis, prepare a written report which shall include

sample – only

information relating to a) the utilization of all medical services provided for Members enrolled in each Participating Physician Practice, including but not limited to, hospital, referral and ancillary services, but excluding prescription drug costs; and b) amounts paid by _____ for claims for such medical services in accordance herewith.

_____ shall then establish budgeted cost targets based on the actual costs of the above medical services provided by all Participating Physicians engaged in Family Practice, Internal Medicine, and Pediatrics Practices.

4.2.4.   Accounting and Distribution. On a quarterly basis, _____ will provide Physician an accounting of his/her eligibility to receive a distribution from the Medical Management Fund with such accounting to be provided no later than one hundred twenty (120) days from the close of the previous accounting period. Distributions shall then be made to each Physician experiencing a favorable variance in net PMPM costs of medical services provided by that Physician compared to the budgeted PMPM cost targets established by _____. The amount of the distribution will be determined by _____, based on the size of the variance, with a maximum distribution of two hundred percent (200%) of the amount credited to the Medical Management Fund for Physician for the quarter.

4.2.5.   Per Member Maximum. The maximum aggregate medical expenses to be tabulated against the targeted medical expenses shall be fifteen thousand dollars ($15,000) per member-per year (POMPEII) exclusive of prescription drug costs.

4.2.6.   Third Party Recoveries. All Coordination of Benefits and Subrogation recoveries pertaining to services performed by Physician or to referral services rendered to Physicians' Members will be credited to the Medical Management Fund, upon receipt of payment.

4.3   Retroactive Member Cancellations and Additions

4.3.1.   Cancellations. If a Member's eligibility has been canceled retroactively, _____ may deduct up to three (3) months Primary Physician Capitation payments to Physician and credit to the Medical Management Fund previously made _____ in respect of such Member from the current payments to, and credits on behalf of, Physician. Physician may bill such _____ Member for services rendered during the period of ineligibility. This activity does not constitute a violation of the provisions of Section 5.3. hereof.

4.3.2.   Additions. If a Member's eligibility has been added retroactively for more than three (3) months, _____ will make capitation payments to Physician and credit the Medical Management Fund for a period not to exceed three (3) months. _____ shall pay Physician for Medical Services provided by Physician during the eligibility period prior to the period for which retroactive payment was made by paying Physician on a fee-for-service basis per Appendix E for applicable services rendered to the Member for the period involved.

4.4. Medical Executive Committee

4.4.1. _____ shall establish a Medical Executive Committee made up of selected physicians, medical professionals and _____ management staff. Voting members of the Committee shall be physicians. The Medical Executive Committee will advise _____ senior management in all matters pertaining to the professional health care provided to Members based upon reports and recommendations from the appropriate staff departments and/or committees. The Medical Executive Committee's responsibilities shall include, but not be limited to, initiation of or participation in the corrective action process or review of measures to ensure ____ ical conduct and competent clinical care are provided to all Members and to ensure the coordination and implementation of clinical protocols and guidelines for the provision of medical services to Members.

5. PHYSICIAN SERVICES TO MEMBERS

5.1. Services Provided and Arranged by Primary Care Physician. Physician shall provide or arrange for and authorize as set forth herein those services covered in the _____ Subscription Agreement. Final determination of Member eligibility and payment of services from the Medical Management Fund shall be made at the- sole discretion of _____. Physician shall abide by all provisions of the _____ Subscription Agreement, which may be amended from time to time, and which is incorporated herein by reference.

5.2. Office Location. Physician shall provide Medical Services to Members at the office location(s) described in Appendix A.

5.3. NAIC Sole Source of Payments Clause. Physician agrees and warrants that in no event, including, but not limited to nonpayment, _____ insolvency or breach of this Agreement, shall Physician bill, charge, collect a deposit from, seek compensation, remuneration or reimbursement from, or have any recourse against Members or persons acting on their behalf for services listed in this Agreement. This provision shall not prohibit collection of supplemental charges or co-payments on _____'s behalf made in accordance with the terms of the _____ Subscription Agreement pertaining to the Member. Physician further agrees that (1) the holdharmless provision and warranty herein shall survive the termination of this Agreement regardless of the cause giving rise to the termination and that (2) this holdharmless provision and warranty supersedes any oral or written contrary agreement heretofore entered into between Physician and Members or persona acting on their behalf. Any modification, addition, or deletion to the provisions of this Section shall become effective on a date no earlier than fifteen (15) days after the Pennsylvania Commissioner of Insurance has received a report of such proposed changes.

5.4.   Medicare Enrolled Members. If Physician provides services to a Member who is a Medicare enrollee, Physician shall accept the Primary Physician Capitation payment from _____, plus payment from Medicare as complete payment for all Medical Services to Member, for services that are the responsibility of Physician under this Agreement.

5.5.   Charges for Excluded and/or Non-Covered Services. Physician may charge Members for Medical Services excluded from the Subscription Agreement, or determine not to be covered by Physician.

5.6.   Preferred Providers. Physician shall refer Members to the approved Preferred Providers. In particular cases, other providers may be used with the prior approval of the _____ Medical Director. In cases where the Member is admitted to a non-preferred hospital due to an emergency, Physician shall participate in arranging for transfer of the Member to a Preferred Provider once the Member's medical condition is stable.

5.7.   Consideration of Referral Specialists. Physician shall routinely use referral specialists who agree:

- Not to bill the Member and to send bills for authorized services to _____.

- To cooperate with the _____ Utilization Review and Quality Assurance programs.

- To cooperate with _____ Consumer Affairs Department in resolving Member problems.

- To accept payments by _____ as payment in full for covered services.

- To accept responsible and competitive fees for their services.

- To use _____ Preferred Providers as specified in a list published and amended by _____, from time to time.

- To permit use of generic substitution for those prescriptions where a generic is available unless the referral specialist specifically indicates that a generic is not medically appropriate.

5.8.   Collection of Member Co-payments. Physician shall collect co-payments from Members for those services designated by _____ as requiring a Member co-payment for Physician services.

5.9.   Generic Drugs. Physician shall permit the use of generic substitution for those prescriptions where a generic is available unless the Physician specifically indicates that a generic is not medically appropriate.

6.   INSPECTION OF SERVICES AND FACILITIES

6.1.   Inspection of Services and Facilities. Physician shall permit authorized representatives of _____ and/or authorized representatives of any state or federal supervisory authority or agency to inspect Physician's facilities and to review the records of Medical Services provided to Members.

7.   RECORDS

7.1.   Physician Records and Procedures. Physician shall maintain, at its sole expense, up-to-date records in accordance with accepted professional standards and sound internal control practices. Physician shall retain and provide access to _____ and any governmental agency to said records for not less than three (3) years after the expiration of this Agreement. Physician shall, upon reasonable notice, provide _____ with any such data as may be requested. _____ may provide forms for keeping certain records, which shall be submitted to _____ by Physician on a monthly basis.

7.2.   Physician Reporting. Physician shall:

- Use _____ Encounter Forms and submit such forms to _____, weekly.

- Use _____ authorization procedures for consultant referrals;

- Provide telephone or written notification to _____ about all authorized hospital admissions, prior to or on the day of admission; and

- _____.

7.3.   Quality Assurance and Utilization Review.   Physician shall participate in the _____ Quality Assurance/Utilization Review Process, including prior review by the _____ Medical Director or his/her designee of all elective admissions and elective surgeries, monitoring for appropriate length of stay, discharge planning and the use of appropriate alternatives for hospitalization and shall attend, or cause a physician associated with Physician to attend, _____ quarterly Advisory Medical Council meetings.

      7.4.   Reporting Requirements of Physician. Physician shall give notice to _____ of any action involving Physician's hospital privileges or conditions relating to his/her ability to admit patients to any hospital or inpatient facility; any situation which develops regarding Physician when notice of that situation has been given to the Bureau of Professional and Occupational Affairs or any other licensing agency or board, or any situation involving an investigation or complaint filed by the Bureau of Professional and Occupational Affairs or any other licensing agency or board, regarding a complaint against Physician's license; when a change in Physician's license to practice medicine or osteopathy is affected or any form of reportable discipline is taken against such license; or any lawsuit or claim filed or asserted against Physician alleging professional malpractice, regardless of whether the lawsuit or claim involves a member.

      In any such instance described above, Physician must notify _____ in writing ten (10) days from the date he/she first receives notice, whether written or oral, with the exception of those lawsuits or claims which do not involve a Member, with respect to which Physician has thirty (30) days to notify _____.

      7.5.   Conflict of Interest. Physician shall report to _____ any transactions in connection with Physician's obligation under this Agreement, with any provider or entity in which Physician has a financial interest.

      8.   STANDARDS

      8.1.   Standards of Care. Physician shall cooperate with _____ in developing written reports on the quality of the Medical Services rendered by Physician, including various techniques developed by Physician and _____ to assure high quality medical services. Physician together with other physicians associated with _____ and/or an outside professional medical organization, society, or university, will establish a mechanism to provide for an external audit of Physician. The findings regarding Physician shall be confidential between _____ and any supervisory authority or agency and Physician. Such external audits are not intended to be punitive, but are to provide means of assuring the quality of medical care. Physician will have the responsibility of implementing any needed changes cited in such audits. The cost of such audits shall be borne by _____; any time spent by Physician in complying herewith shall not be reimbursed. _____ and Physician further agree to jointly develop methods, procedures and techniques designed to educate all Members receiving health care hereunder, regarding the proper utilization of Medical Services.

8.2.   Principles of Practice. Physician shall abide by the Principles of Practice as adopted and amended by _____.

8.3.   High Quality Cost Effective Care. Physician shall provide and arrange for high quality, cost effective medical care in accordance with _____ policies.

8.4.   Service Standards. Treat Members with the same levels of courtesy and respect accorded all other patients of Physician, and comply with the Member Service Standards set forth in the _____ Principles of Practice.

8.5.   Hospital Admitting Privileges. Physician must maintain admitting privileges at one or more participating hospitals.

9.   INSURANCE

9.1.   Liability Insurance Requirements. Physician shall ensure that Physician and each physician associated with Physician who provides services under this Agreement to _____ Members carries at his/her own expense, or is covered under policies provided by Physician at its sole expense:

- Liability insurance of at least one million dollars ($1,000,000) per person/per occurrence and, at least, three million dollars ($3,000,000) in the annual aggregate insuring against professional errors and omissions (malpractice) in providing medical services under the terms of this Agreement, and if available, without additional expense to the physician, naming as an additional co-insured; and _____.

  Insurance which has the effect of providing reasonable and adequate coverage in the event of personal injury on or about the premises of Physician.

- Insurance which has the effect of providing reasonable and adequate coverage in the event of personal injury on or about the premises of Physician.

Physician at its sole expense, if any, shall cause certificates of insurance or verifications of required coverages containing a 30-day notice of cancellation to _____ to be issued to _____ for all coverages listed herein and for subsequent renewals of all required coverages.

sample – only

9.2.   "Tail Coverage." If any of the insurance coverages described in Section 8.1. are provided through "claims made" rather than "occurrence" forms, then Physician shall provide, or ensure that the physicians associated with it provide "tail coverage" in the amounts described in Section 8.1. upon the termination or expiration of this Agreement or the termination or expiration of such physicians' association with Physician.

10.   SOLICITATION OF MEMBERS

10.1.   Solicitation of Members to Change. During the term of this Agreement or any renewal thereof, and for a period of one year from the date of termination, neither Physician nor any physician associated with Physician shall.., within the Service Area of the Plan, advise or counsel any _____ member to end enrollment with _____ and will not solicit any such Member to become enrolled with any other health maintenance organization or other hospitalization or medical payment plan or insurance policy.

11.   TERM AND TERMINATION

11.1.   Notice Required to Terminate Agreement. This Agreement will commence on the date set forth in the Preamble of this Agreement and shall continue in effect indefinitely unless or until either party notifies the other in writing not less than ninety (90) days prior to the anniversary of the effective date that it desires to terminate the Agreement on such anniversary date. This Agreement may be terminated at any time upon the mutual consent of the parties with sixty (60) days prior written notice. In addition, under the circumstances specified in Section 12.3, Physician may terminate this Agreement upon the effective date of any proposed amendment to this Agreement provided Physician shall have given _____ at least sixty (60) days written notice of such termination.

11.2.   Termination of Agreement for Cause. Either party may terminate this Agreement at any time for cause upon delivery of written notice, in the event of the following:

11.2.1.   Material Default. The other party shall materially default in the performance of a provision of this Agreement or any other agreements referred to herein and such default shall continue for a period of thirty (30) days after the mailing of written notice of the defaulting party stating the specific default.

11.2.2.   Bankruptcy and Other Insolvency. The other party shall apply for or consent to the appointment of a receiver, trustee or liquidator of all or a substantial part of its assets, file a voluntary petition in bankruptcy, or admit in writing its inability to pay its debts as they become due, make a general assignment for the benefit of creditors, file a petition or an answer seeking reorganization or arrangement with creditors or to take advantage of an insolvency law, or if an order, judgment or decree shall be entered by a court of competent jurisdiction, or the application or a liquidator of all or a substantial part of its assets, creditor, adjudicating such a party a bankrupt or insolvent or approving a petition seeking reorganization of the party or appointment of a receiver, trustee or liquidator of all or a substantial part of its assets.

11.2.3.   Loss of License. The other party loses its state license to operate an HMO or to practice medicine or osteopathy.

11.3.   Notice to Members about Termination of Agreement. _____ shall be solely responsible for notifying Members that this Agreement has been terminated by Physician or _____.

11.4.   Rights of Parties Upon Termination. Upon the expiration or termination of this Agreement:

Physician shall turn over to _____ - and shall make available to _____ such information and records as may be requested.

Physician shall transfer copies of _____ Member records to Participating Physician subsequently chosen by Members transferring out of Physician's practice.

Physician shall remain obligated to provide Medical Services to any Member who is at the time of said expiration or termination a registered bed patient at a hospital until such Member's discharge from the hospital and _____ will reimburse Physician for such Medical Services at the fee schedule being used by _____ at the time of service.

11.5.   Danger to Health or Safety of Members. _____ may suspend this Agreement immediately whenever _____ believes that there is clear and convincing evidence that the health or safety of _____ Members is endangered by actions of the Physician, or agents or employees of the Physician. In the event that such condition is continuing and remains unresolved with a reasonable satisfaction to _____ for a period of thirty (30) days, _____ may terminate this Agreement effective immediately upon notification to the Physician.

12.   ASSIGNMENT

12.1.   Assignment of Agreement. This Agreement, being intended to secure the personal services of Physician, shall not be assigned or transferred by Physician. The execution of this Agreement by Physician constitutes Physician's prior written consent to the Assignment of this Agreement by _____ to a Physician Network, to be created as soon as practicable after the effective date of this Agreement and to consist, in whole or in part, of Participating Physicians affiliated with

_____.

13.   AMENDMENTS

13.1.   Amendment by Mutual Written Agreement. This Agreement may be amended at any time by the mutual written agreement of Physician and _____. This Agreement is subject to all rules and regulations promulgated at any time by any state or federal regulatory agency or authority having supervisory authority over _____, and this Agreement shall be deemed to be amended to conform therewith at all times.

13.2.   Subscription Agreement. If any provision of this Agreement is inconsistent, or in conflict with, any Subscription Agreement in effect from time to time which sets forth the rights of Members, the Subscription Agreement then in effect shall take precedence.

13.3.   Amendments by _____ shall have the right to promulgate amendments to this Agreement and the Appendices to this Agreement by notifying Physician at least ninety (90) days prior to the effective date of the amendment. If Physician has not given notice of termination of this Agreement at least sixty (60) days prior to the effective date of the amendment, Physician will be deemed to have agreed to the amendment and will be bound by it.

14.   SEVERABILITY

14.1.1   Severability. If any one or more of the provisions contained in this Agreement shall for any reason be held to be invalid, illegal or unenforceable in any respect, such invalidity, illegality or unenforceability shall not affect any other provisions of this Agreement, and this Agreement shall be construed as if such invalid, illegal or unenforceable provision had never been contained herein.

15.MISCELLANEOUS

15.1.   Binding Effect Agreement. This Agreement shall inure to the benefit of and be binding upon the parties hereto, their employees, successors and permitted assigns. Except with respect to Section 4.3, this Agreement is not intended to be a third-party beneficiary contract or to confer any rights on any third person.

15.2.   Notice. Any notice required by this Agreement shall be given by registered or certified mail, addressed to the party to whom such notice is intended to be given, at the last known address of that party's principal place of business.

15.3.   Governing Law. All matters affecting the interpretation of this Agreement and the rights and obligations of the parties hereto shall be governed by and construed in accordance with the laws of the (State of Commonwealth) of _____.

15.4.   Waiver. The failure of any party to insist upon the strict performance of any provision of this Agreement shall not be deemed to be a waiver of any breach of this Agreement or the right to insist upon strict performance of such provision at any future time.

15.5   Entire Agreement. This Agreement and the appendices and attachments hereto, as modified by the Subscription Agreement, is the entire Agreement between the parties and supersedes any and all prior agreements between _____ and Physician or any predecessor of either party with the other.

15.6.   Authority to Sign Agreement. The person signing this Agreement on behalf of Physician represents and warrants that such person is duly authorized and empowered to execute this Agreement on behalf of the Physician.

15.7.   Signatures. Physician warrants that each partner of the partnership, or professional association, shareholder of the professional corporation, or employee of same who is a doctor of medicine or (specialty) _____ has consented to this Agreement by affixing his or her signature below.

IN WITNESS WHEREOF, this Agreement is executed by — _____ and Physician, as of the date and year set forth above.

_____

_____ CORPORATION:

By: _____

Title: _____

PHYSICIAN:

_____   _____
Print Name   Signature

PARTNERS OR SHAREHOLDERS—OR PHYSICIAN-EMPLOYEES
        Print: Signature:

_____   _____

_____   _____

_____   _____

/eb

<u>sample – only</u>

APPENDIX - A

PHYSICIAN agrees to accept at least _____ (___) members.

OFFICE LOCATIONS:

PHYSICIAN shall provide Medical Services pursuant to the terms of this Agreement, at the following location(s):

LOCATION 1

_____
Practice Name

_____
Address

_____
City - State - Zip

Phone: _____

LOCATION 2

_____
Practice Name

_____
Address

_____
City - State - Zip

Phone: _____

LOCATION 3

_____
Practice Name

_____
Address

_____
City - State - Zip

Phone: _____

LOCATION 4

_____
Practice Name

_____
Address

_____
City - State - Zip

Phone: _____

sample – only

APPENDIX - B

PHYSICIAN COMPENSATION

Member Age	Sex	Primary Physician Capitation Fund: Per Member/per Month
0–23 months	Male	$ 39.54
	Female	39.54
2–4 years	Male	13.99
	Female	13.99
5–19 years	Male	9.72
	Female	9.72
20–44 years	Male	9.32
	Female	14.90
45–64 years	Male	14.90
	Female	18.77
65 years or older	Male	16.49
	Female	16.49

APPENDIX - C

I. Examples of Services Covered from Primary Physician Capitation Fund

- Office Visits (includes medical supplies)

- hour-per-day availability or backup

- Physical Exams

- Injections (excluding cost of allergy serums)

- Immunizations

- All Level I Laboratory Service

- Home Visits

- Hospital Visits

- Nursing Home Visits

- Surgical Procedures Performed in Physician's Office

- Health Education in Physician's Office

- Nutrition Counseling in Physician's Office

- Mental Health Counseling in Physician's Office

sample – only

APPENDIX - D

The Service Area of the Plan is _____
(County/Commonwealth) and such other areas as the Plan may, from time
to time designate.

APPENDIX - E

FEE SCHEDULE FOR OTHER PRODUCTS

Medical Services and surgical procedures rendered in the Physician's office will be paid according to the _____ fee schedule, as established from time to time.

SAMPLE
PHYSICIAN AGREEMENT AMENDMENT

The Physician Agreement dated as of this _____
day of _____, 19_____, between _____
("Physician"), and _____ of (county/commonwealth)
_____ of _____ (state), is hereby amended,
as follows:

_____ operates a Health Maintenance Organization
in the Service Area and_____, a Preferred Provider
Organization ("PPO"), is subcontracting with _____ for
Physician services to be provided to its members.

The parties hereby agree, as follows:

Physician agrees to participate in the PPO. PPO is a Non-Risk
Assuming Preferred Provider Organization which contracts directly with
"Self-Funded Entities" (e.g., employers, unions, associations, etc.) who are
responsible for funding of medical claims.

PPO may also contract with an "Insurance Carrier" to administer
their PPO arrangement. When _____ contracts with an
Insurance Carrier, said carrier is responsible for funding of medical claims.

As a participant in the PPO, Physician agrees to maintain
responsibility for the Quality Assurance and delivery system controls
outlined in the Physician Agreement. Physician shall coordinate and provide
care for PPO members in the same manner as provided to
_____ members.

Physician further agrees to the following:

1.   Physician shall participate in the activities of, and agree to
be bound by the policies adopted by and the decisions of the HMO's Quality
Assurance and Utilization Management Committees as applicable to PPO
members. Such activities include but are not limited to credentialing,
maintaining hospital privileges and participating in office audits; and,

sample – only

2.   Physician shall cooperate with and abide by the decisions of the HMO's Member Grievance System as applicable to PPO members; and,

3.   Physician shall provide access to member medical records to the PPO and/or Department of Health when such access is required for the purpose of quality oversight and grievance resolution; and,

4.   PPO shall retain the right to immediately suspend or terminate Physician's participation in the PPO if Physician's license to practice medicine is suspended or revoked, or if PPO determines that said Physician, in treating PPO members failed to act professionally or has or may act in any manner which may harm PPO members.

For services provided to Point of Service PPO Members, _____ will reimburse physician according to the currently applicable Primary Physician POS PPO capitation payment schedule. In addition, physician may collect applicable co-payments from those members.

Subject to the aforesaid amendments, all other provisions of the original Physician Agreement remain in full force and effect.

This Amendment is effective the _____ day of _____, 19____.

_____   _____
By: President & Chief Executive Officer

(Tax I.D. _____)

sample – only

MEDICARE AMENDMENT

THIS MEDICARE AMENDMENT (this "Amendment") is made this
_____ day of _____, 19_____, by and between
_____ operating as a managed care organization
("MCO"), and _____, P.C. ("Physician").

WHEREAS, MCO operates a health maintenance organization (the
"HMO") that is licensed in the _____
(county/commonwealth) of _____ (state); and

WHEREAS, MCO shall enter into a risk contract with HCFA
(hereinafter defined) pursuant to which MCO shall offer the Medicare Plan
(hereinafter defined) to Medicare eligible individuals; and

WHEREAS, MCO and Physician entered into an agreement (the
"Physician Agreement") whereby Physician agreed to provide professional
services to members of the HMO; and

WHEREAS, MCO and Physician desire to amend the Physician
Agreement pursuant to which amendment Physician shall participate in the
Medicare Plan and provide Medicare Covered Services (hereinafter defined)
to Medicare Covered Individuals (hereinafter defined).

NOW THEREFORE, the parties hereto, intending to be legally bound
hereby agree, as follows:

WHEREAS, MCO and Physician entered into an agreement (the
"Physician Agreement") whereby Physician agreed

1.   **DEFINITIONS**

The terms listed below, whether used in the singular or plural, shall
have the meanings set forth below when used in this Amendment.
        1.1.   "Evidence of Coverage" shall mean the contract, as
amended from time to time, between MCO and a Medicare Covered
Individual which sets forth the contractual rights and obligations of the
parties thereto and which describes the Medicare Covered Services,
requirements, limitations and exclusions of the managed care benefit plan
set forth therein.

sample – only

1.2.   "HCFA" shall mean the Health Care Financing Administration of the United States of America.

1.3.   "HCFA Contract" shall mean the contract entered into by and between MCO and HCFA, as amended from time to time, pursuant to which MCO shall offer the Medicare Plan.

1.4.   "Medicare" shall mean the Medicare program administered by HCFA.

1.5.   "Medicare Covered Individual" shall mean an individual eligible to receive Medicare Covered Services.

1.6.   "Medicare Covered Services" shall mean those Medically Necessary health care services and supplies described in the Evidence of Coverage, as amended, under which the Medicare Covered Individual being treated is covered.

1.7.   "Medicare Participating Provider" shall mean a licensed physician, hospital, skilled nursing facility, home health care agency, or other provider of health care services who has entered into a written agreement with MCO to provide Medicare Covered Services to Medicare Covered Individuals.

Unless otherwise defined herein, capitalized terms shall have the meanings set forth in the Physician Agreement.

2.   MEDICARE COVERED SERVICES

Physician shall provide Medicare Covered Services to Medicare Covered Individuals on a twenty-four (24) hour per day, seven (7) day per week basis, in accordance with this Amendment and the Physician Agreement. Notwithstanding the foregoing, in the event that Physician cannot provide such coverage on a twenty-four (24) hour per day, seven (7) days per week basis, Physician may arrange for a physician who is a Medicare Participating Provider to provide coverage on Physician's behalf so long as Physician retains primary responsibility for Medicare Covered Individuals' care.

Physician shall refer Medicare Covered Individuals only to other Medicare Participating Providers to receive Medicare Covered Services, unless a referral to a non-Medicare Participating Provider is authorized by MCO's Medical Director.

3.   **NON-DISCRIMINATION**

Physician shall provide Medicare Covered Services to Medicare
Covered Individuals in the same manner as professional services are
provided to all other Physician patients according to the severity of the
medical need and the availability of personnel, equipment and necessary
facilities; provided, however, in no event shall Physician provide Medicare
Covered Services to Medicare Covered Individuals in accordance with
standards less than those standards set forth in the Physician Agreement,
this Amendment and the prevailing standards in the community in which
Physician provides services.

Physician shall not discriminate against Medicare Covered
Individuals on the basis of age, race, color, creed, religion, sex, sexual
preference, national origin, health status, income level or on the basis that
they are members of a prepaid health care plan or a Medicare beneficiary.
Physician shall not refuse to provide Medicare Covered Services to, or
attempt to discharge, Medicare Covered Individuals on the basis of credit
history.

Further, Physician shall not refuse to accept Medicare Covered
Individuals as patients so long as Physician accepts patients who are
insured under any other third party Medicare risk insurance plan.

4.   **ADVANCE DIRECTIVES**

Physician shall document in each Medicare Covered Individual's
medical record whether the Medicare Covered Individual has executed an
advance directive. Physician shall not condition treatment or otherwise
discriminate on the basis of whether a Medicare Covered Individual has
executed an advance directive.

5.   **ADMINISTRATIVE SERVICES**

MCO shall perform the administrative, claims processing,
marketing, enrollment, quality management and utilization management
functions that are required of an HMO and a HCFA risk reimbursement
contractor. MCO shall make every reasonable effort to ensure that persons
enrolled in the Medicare Plan are eligible to participate in the Medicare

sample – only

Plan; however, MCO assumes no liability hereunder or otherwise for payment for services rendered to any persons that determined later not to be eligible to participate in the Medicare Plan.

6. PHYSICIAN REMUNERATION

In consideration of Physician's agreement to perform Medicare Covered Services in accordance with this Amendment, MCO shall pay Physician for Medicare Covered Services performed as set forth in Appendix A, attached hereto and made a part hereof.

Physician understands and agrees that payment to Physician for performance of Medicare Covered Services shall be subject to the authorization and eligibility procedures set forth in the Physician Agreement. Physician further understands and agrees that payment to Physician for Medicare Covered Services (whether capitation or fee-for-service payments), including amounts recovered by Physician through coordination of benefits, shall constitute payment in full for all professional services for which Physician bills, whether professional or technical in nature and shall satisfy in full MCO's payment obligation hereunder. Upon such payment, Physician shall have no further recourse against MCO or a Medicare Covered Individual unless otherwise permitted under this Amendment or the Physician Agreement.

In no event shall Physician seek payment from any person other than MCO for Medicare Covered Services rendered to Medicare Covered Individuals; provided, however, Physician may seek payment from a patient for professional services that are not Medicare Covered Services so long as Physician advises the Covered Individual of his/her payment responsibility prior to rendering any such professional services.

7. COMPLIANCE WITH GOVERNMENT REQUIREMENTS

Physician shall comply with all applicable requirements, laws, rules and regulations of HCFA, any other federal agency and state agencies of the state in which Physician practices, including without limitation, requirements that shall cause or require MCO to amend the terms and conditions of this Amendment. Physician understands and agrees that

HCFA and the appropriate state agencies may change or add to such requirements, laws, rules and regulations from time to time. Physician further agrees to comply with any such changes and additions.

8.   **RELEASE OF INFORMATION**

In addition to complying with the disclosure and other information requirements set forth in the Physician Agreement, Physician agrees to release to MCO all information requested by MCO for the purpose of enabling MCO to comply with its obligations to provide information to HCFA under the HCFA Contract or applicable law.

Physician further agrees, on behalf of itself and its subcontractors, to provide to MCO and HCFA full and complete information as to : (i) the ownership of a subcontractor with whom Physician has had business transactions in an aggregate amount in excess of $25,000 during the twelve months ending on the date of the applicable HCFA request for information from Physician or MCO, and (ii) any significant business transactions between Physician and any wholly-owned supplier or between Physician and any subcontractor during the five year period ending on the date of the applicable HCFA request for information from Physician or MCO. The required information must be provided in the manner required under Section 1866(b)(2)(c)(ii) of the Social Security Act, as amended.

Physician understands and agrees that in no event shall MCO or HCFA be required to reimburse Physician for expenses related to providing copies of patient records or documents provided to (i) HCFA; (ii) MCO pursuant to a request from HCFA or other state or federal agency; or (iii) MCO in order to assist MCO in making a determination regarding payment due hereunder.

9.   **HCFA INSPECTION**

Physician shall permit authorized representatives of HCFA to inspect Physician's facilities and to review: (i) the medical records of Medicare Covered Individuals, (ii) records of Physician relating to the provision of Medicare Covered Services, and (iii) any additional records relating in any way to the subject matter of this Amendment. Physician shall

sample – only

cooperate fully with HCFA in any such inspections, which inspections Physician agrees may be conducted by HCFA or any other federal or state agency without prior notice to Physician.

10.   NON-DISCLOSURE OF HCFA RECORDS

Physician agrees to establish and maintain procedures and controls so that no information contained in its records or obtained from HCFA or from others in carrying out the terms of this Amendment shall be used or disclosed by Physician, its agents, officers or employees except as provided in Section 1106 of the Social Security Act and regulations prescribed thereunder.

11.   ELIGIBILITY TO PROVIDE SERVICES TO MEDICARE RECIPIENTS

Physician represents and warrants that Physician is, and shall continue to be, eligible to participate in Medicare. Physician shall promptly notify MCO if Physician, or any physician practicing in association with Physician, is suspended or terminated from participation in Medicare or the medical assistance program of any state. Upon such suspension or termination, MCO shall be entitled to terminate this Amendment and the Physician Agreement upon sixty (60) days prior written notice to Physician.

Physician understands and agrees that MCO shall not be liable for payment (whether capitation, fee-for-service or other payment method) for Medicare Covered Services rendered by Physician from and after the date that Physician is suspended or terminated from participation in Medicare. Further, Physician shall refund any and all amounts paid by MCO for Medicare Covered Services rendered by Physician from and after the date Physician is suspended or terminated from participating in Medicare.

12.   ADDITIONAL PHYSICIANS/PRACTICES

12.1.   Physicians. Whenever one or more additional physicians are to begin practicing as part of Physician's practice (referred to herein as an "Additional Physician"), whether as a result of a Change of Control Event (hereinafter defined) or otherwise, Physician shall give MCO at least thirty (30) days prior written notice of the intended addition of any such Additional

Physician(s). Physician acknowledges that such Additional Physician(s) shall not automatically be deemed to be part of Physician under the Physician Agreement or this Amendment, but that the addition of such Additional Physician(s) to the Physician Agreement and this Amendment shall be subject to the provisions of this Section 12 and to MCO's standard credentialing process.

12.2.   Practices. Whenever Physician is to acquire one or more additional practices (referred to herein as an "Additional Practice") and one or more Additional Physicians are to begin practicing as part of Physician's practice, whether as a result of a Change of Control Event or otherwise Physician shall give MCO at least thirty (30) days prior written notice of the intended addition of such Additional Practice(s) and Additional Physician(s). Physician acknowledges that the Additional Physician(s) in such Additional Practice(s) shall not automatically be deemed to be part of Physician under the Physician Agreement or this Amendment, but that the addition of such Additional Practice(s) and Additional Physician(s) associated therewith to the Physician Agreement and this Amendment shall be subject to the provisions of this Section 12 and to MCO's standard credentialing process.

12.3.   Change of Control. Physician acknowledges that the relationship between MCO and Physician is a personal one, and that MCO's decision to enter into the Physician Agreement and this Amendment with Physician is based on an assumption that the current ownership and control of Physician will not change. Accordingly, Physician agrees that MCO will be given at least thirty (30) days prior written notice of any of the events listed immediately below (each a "Change of Control Event"):

12.3.1   - any merger or consolidation of Physician or any physician practice associated with Physician (collectively for purposes of this Section 12 only, "Physician") with any other corporation, partnership, practice, person or entity of any nature ("Person"), including by way of the purchase of any capital stock or assets of any Person;

12.3.2.   - sale, lease or other transfer of any of Physician's assets to any Person, other than sales or leases of assets in the ordinary course of business;

12.3.3.   - sale or other transfer of any of the stock in any professional corporation in which Physician is a shareholder or that employs Physician, issuance of any additional shares of stock in such corporation, or redemption or purchase of any shares of stock of such corporation;

sample – only

12.3.4.　　- sales, purchase, or other transfer of any partnership interest in a medical partnership in which Physician owns a partnership interest or that employs Physician;

12.3.5.　　- entry into any management contract permitting a third party management rights with respect to Physician's practice; or a change in the Tax I.D. Number under which Physician collects payment for professional services.

12.4.　　Breach. Physician agrees that in no event, including but not limited to nonpayment by MCO, insolvency of MCO or breach of this Amendment, shall Physician bill, charge, collect a deposit from, seek compensation, remuneration or reimbursement from, or have any recourse against a Medicare Covered Individual, or a person acting on behalf of a Medicare Covered Individual, for Medicare Covered Services provided pursuant to this Amendment. This Section 13.1 does not prohibit Physician from collecting Deductibles or Copayments, as specifically provided in the applicable Evidence of Coverage, or fees-for-professional services that are not Medicare Covered Services delivered on a fee-for-service basis to Medicare Covered Individuals, so long as, in the case of professional services that are not Medicare Covered Services, Physician advises the Medicare Covered Individual of his/her payment responsibility prior to rendering any such professional services.

13.　　**NO BALANCE BILLING/CONTINUATION OF BENEFITS**

13.1.　　No Balance Billing. Physician agrees that in no event, including but not limited to nonpayment by MCO, insolvency of MCO or breach of this Amendment, shall Physician bill, charge, collect a deposit from, seek compensation, remuneration or reimbursement from, or have any recourse against a Medicare Covered Individual, or a person acting on behalf of a Medicare Covered Individual, for Medicare Covered Services provided pursuant to this Amendment. This Section 13.1 does not prohibit Physician from collecting Deductibles or Copayments, as specifically provided in the applicable Evidence of Coverage, or fees-for professional services that are not Medicare Covered Services delivered on a fee-for-service basis to Medicare Covered Individuals so long as, in the case of professional services that are not Medicare Covered Services, Physician advises the Medicare Covered Individual of his/her payment responsibility prior to rendering any such professional services.

14.　　**GROUP PRACTICE**

In the event that Physician is a professional corporation, association, partnership or other corporate entity, Physician hereby represents and warrants to MCO that: (i) each physician that provides Medicare Covered Services on behalf of Physician is licensed to practice medicine or _____ (specialty) in the _____ (county/commonwealth) of _____ (state); (ii) each physician that provides Medicare Covered Services on behalf of Physician has agreed to be bound by the terms and conditions of the Physician Agreement and this Amendment; and (iii) the person signing this Amendment on behalf of Physician is duly authorized and empowered to execute and deliver this Amendment on behalf of Physician. Notwithstanding the foregoing, Physician understands and agrees that a physician may not provide Medicare Covered Services on behalf of Physicians unless and until such physician has been accepted as a Participating Physician by MCO, which acceptance shall be in writing. In the event that Physician is a professional corporation, association, partnership or other corporate entity, a list setting forth, among other things, the physicians that provide professional services on behalf of Physician as of the date of this Amendment shall be attached to this Amendment as Appendix B.

15.   **EFFECT OF AMENDMENT**

This Amendment sets forth the terms and conditions under which Physician shall render Medicare Covered Services to Medicare Covered Individuals; provided, however, any matter relating to the provision of Medicare Covered Services to Medicare covered Individuals that is not specifically provided for in this Amendment shall be governed by the Physician Agreement, in which matter the Physician Agreement shall be interpreted and read as though Medicare Covered Individuals are Members. Notwithstanding the foregoing, in the event of a conflict between the terms and conditions of the Physician Agreement and this Amendment, the terms and conditions of this Amendment shall control. This Amendment in no way affects the terms and conditions of the Physician Agreement; provided, however, the Physician Agreement shall terminate immediately in the event that this Amendment is terminated.

16.   **ASSIGNMENT**

This Amendment is intended to secure the personal services of Physician, and therefore, neither this Amendment nor any of the obligations hereunder may be assigned or transferred in any manner without the prior written consent of MCO, which consent may be withheld in MCO's sole and absolute discretion. Any such attempted assignment without the consent of MCO shall be null and void. MCO may assigned this Amendment upon thirty (30) days written prior notice to Physician.

17.   **GOVERNING LAW**

This Amendment shall be governed by and construed in accordance with the laws of the _____ (county/commonwealth) of _____ (state), without regard to its choice of law provisions.

sample – only

18.   **ENTIRE AGREEMENT AND AMENDMENT**

This Amendment constitutes the entire understanding of the parties hereto with regard to the subject matter hereof and supersedes any and all written or oral agreements, representations, or understandings. MCO shall have the right to promulgate amendments to this Amendment by notifying Physician at least sixty (60) days prior to the effective date of the amendment.

Physician may terminate this Amendment upon Physician's receipt of such notice of amendment, by notifying MCO in writing of such termination; provided, however, if MCO has not received notice of such termination at least thirty (30) days prior to the effective date of the amendment, Physician will be deemed to have agreed to the amendment and will be bound thereby. No other modifications, discharges, amendment or alterations shall be effective unless evidenced by an instrument in writing, signed by Physician and MCO.

IN WITNESS WHEREOF, this Agreement has been duly executed by Physician and the duly authorized representative of MCO, as of the date first written above.

PHYSICIAN: MANAGED CARE ORGANIZATION:

By: _____   By: _____

Print Name: _____   Print Name: _____

Print Title: _____   Print Title: _____

Tax I.D. #: _____

APPENDIX A

PAYMENT PROVISIONS

1.   **BASE PAY**

1.1.   Capitation. MCO shall make monthly payments to Physician equal to the number of Covered Individuals enrolled in Physician's practice by the first day of the previous calendar month multiplied by the appropriate dollar amounts specified in Schedule 1 attached hereto and made a part hereof. (Amounts paid to Physician pursuant to the foregoing sentence are referred to herein as the "Primary Physician Capitation").

sample – only

1.2.   Payment Schedule. MCO shall make payments to Physician for covered Services rendered, in the case of the Primary Physician Capitation, on or before the tenth (10th) working day of each month and, in the case of fee-for-service payments, at the rates provided in the applicable MCO Medicare fee schedule within thirty (30) days of MCO's receipt of a properly completed claim form. Such payment periods may be extended if additional time is required to investigate whether the number and type of Covered Individuals reported by Physician is accurate, the services rendered are Covered Services or MCO, or another entity is responsible for payment for such Covered Services.

1.3.   Retroactively. If a Covered Individual's eligibility has been canceled retroactively, MCO may deduct from payments due Physician an amount equal to the Primary Physician Capitation payments previously paid to Physician for Covered Services rendered to such Covered Individual after the date of the retroactive cancellation; provided, however, such amount shall not exceed an amount equal to three (3) months of Primary Physician Capitation payments for such Covered Services. Physician may bill such Covered Individual for services rendered during such period of ineligibility, which billing shall not constitute a violation of this Agreement. If a Covered Individual's enrollment in Physician's practice has been added retroactively for three (3) or more months, MCO shall make a Primary Physician Capitation payment equal to three months of Primary Physician Capitation payments for such Covered Individual. Physician must notify MCO immediately if a Medicare covered Individual requests that Physician provide Medicare Covered Services and the Medicare Covered Individual is not yet enrolled in Physician's practice. The foregoing financial terms and conditions shall be Physician's sole and exclusive remedy if Physician provides Covered Services for a Medicare Covered Individual who is not enrolled in Physician's practice.

2.   **INCENTIVE PAYMENT**

In addition to the Primary Physician Capitation, Physician may be entitled to receive the incentive payments described in detail below:

2.1.   Eligibility. MCO wishes to allow Participating Physicians to participate in the savings enjoyed by MCO due to Participating Physicians' efficient management of the Covered Services provided to Covered Individuals. (For purposes of this Section 2 only, a Covered Individual is sometimes referred to as a Member.) MCO shall make an annual incentive payment to Physician if: (i) the contract by and between MCO and Physician providing for Physician's performance of covered Services was in effect each of the twelve (12) months in the calendar year preceding the distribution; (ii) Physician provided Covered Services to Covered Individuals during such calendar year, in accordance with such contract; and (iii) Physician meets the conditions set forth below.

sample – only

2.2.   Calculation of Incentive Payment. If Physician qualifies under Section 2.1 above, MCO shall make an annual payment to Physician in accordance with Section 2.5 below equal to the aggregate amount of payments due under Sections 2.2.1; 2.2.2; and 2.2.3, below.

2.2.1.   Annual Number of Inpatient Bed Days. If the total annual amount of Inpatient Days hereinafter defined for all Covered Individuals enrolled in Physician's practice during the calendar year is less than or equal to the rate of 1,400 Inpatient days per 1,000 Covered Individuals, MCO shall pay Physician an amount equal to the applicable PMPM (hereinafter defined) amount set forth in Section I of Schedule 2 attached hereto and made a part hereof.

2.2.2.   Average Length of Stay. If the annual average number of Inpatient Days per each admission for each Medicare Covered Individual enrolled in Physician's practice during the calendar year is less than six (6) Inpatient Days (sometimes referred to herein as the "Average Length of Stay" or "ALOS"), MCO shall pay Physician an amount equal to the applicable PMPM amount set forth in Section II of Schedule 2.

2.2.3.   Outpatient Services. If the total annual amount paid by MCO for Outpatient Services (hereinafter defined) received by all Medicare Covered Individuals enrolled in Physician's practice during a calendar year is no more than Ten Percent (10%) above Physician's Target Number (hereinafter defined), MCO shall pay Physician an amount equal to the Applicable percentage amount set forth in Section III of Schedule 2 multiplied by $.50 PMPM. Notwithstanding the foregoing, amounts paid by MCO for Outpatient Services received by each Medicare Covered Individual in a calendar year in excess of $25,000 shall not be included in the calculation of the total annual amount paid by MCO for Outpatient Services received by all Medicare Covered Individuals enrolled in Physician's practice during the calendar year.

2.3   Definitions

2.3.1   "Inpatient Day" shall mean a day that a Covered Individual is receiving Covered Services in a licensed bed operated by an acute care hospital as of the hospital's census taking hour; provided, however, an Inpatient Day at the facilities or departments listed below shall be calculated as a portion of an Inpatient Day as set forth below:

Facility/Department	Portion of Inpatient Day
Skilled Nursing Facility	.25
Mental Health/Chemical Dependency Department	.50
Rehabilitation Department	.70

sample – only

2.3.2   "PMPM" or "Per Member Per Month" shall mean the amount to be paid to Physician, as calculated on a monthly basis, per each Covered Individual enrolled in Physician's practice by the first day of the calendar month.

2.3.3.   "Outpatient Services" shall mean the professional and technical portion of outpatient services received by Covered Individuals enrolled in Physician's practice; provided, however, Outpatient Services shall not include: (i) outpatient services received at a skilled nursing facility or as part of home health care; (ii) home I.V. therapy; (iii) durable medical equipment; (iv) pharmaceuticals; (v) optical services or devices; or (v) dental services or devices.

2.3.4.   "Target Number" shall mean the dollar amount established by MCO, in its sole discretion, which shall represent the recommended total annual dollar amount to be paid by MCO for Outpatient Services received by Covered Individuals enrolled in Physician's practice and shall take into account the age and sex of the Covered Individuals enrolled in Physician's practice.

2.4.   Reporting. On or before the one-hundred twentieth (120th) day following the end of each calendar quarter, MCO shall provide to Physician a report setting forth, among other things, the utilization data described above for the previous calendar quarter and the calendar year-to-date. Such report shall be based upon the utilization data received by MCO on or before the ninetieth (90th) day following the end of each calendar quarter.

2.5.   Distribution. On or before May 1 of each calendar year, MCO shall pay to Physician an amount equal to the aggregate amount of payments due under Sections 2.2.1; 2.2.2; and 2.2.3 above, and based upon the data set forth in the quarterly reports described above.

SCHEDULE 1

CAPITATION RATES

Member Age	$0 Copay		$8 Copay	
	Male	Female	Male	Female
0–64—Base	18.45	28.96	15.93	25.01
65–69—Base	22.33	19.54	19.20	16.80
70–74—Base	26.03	22.12	22.25	18.91
75–84—Base	30.70	25.92	26.38	22.28
85+—Base	33.08	28.76	28.30	24.61

SCHEDULE 2

INCENTIVE RATES

I. INPATIENT DAYS

Inpatient Days per 1,000 Medicare Covered Individuals	PMPM Credit
1,401+	$00.00
1,351–1,400	.19
1,301–1,350	.41
1,251–1,300	.68
1,201–1,250	.98
1,151–1,200	1.31
1,101–1,150	1.80
1,051–1,100	2.36
0–1,050	3.00

II. AVERAGE LENGTH OF STAY

ALOS	PMPM Credit
6.0+	$ 00.00
5.8–5.9	.20
5.6–5.7	.47
5.4–5.5	.82
5.2–5.3	1.25
5.0–5.1	1.76
0–4.9	2.35

sample – only

SCHEDULE 2 - (continued)

III. OUTPATIENT SERVICES

Percentage under Target Number	Percentage Multiplied by $.50 PMPM
10% or more	200%
9–9.9	180
8–8.9	160
7–7.9	140
6–6.9	130
5–5.9	120
4–4.9	115
3–3.9	110
2–2.9	105
0–1.9	100

Percentage over Target Number

0–1.9%	100%
2–2.9	95
3–3.9	90
4–4.9	85
5–5.9	80
6–6.9	70
7–7.9	60
8–8.9	40
9–9.9	20
10% or more	0

Microsoftword-
a:\physagt2.jfm

sample – only

QUESTIONS RELATING TO THE SAMPLE CAPITATED CONTRACT

Many of the 50 questions in the previous chapter would be appropriate to ask when negotiating the sample capitated contract. However, those questions are general in design to assist physicians and their administrators in dealing with most managed care/capitated contracts. Therefore, I have developed a set of specific questions for this sample to give the readers ideas about how to apply the questions from the previous chapter to specific contracts. The following questions are in no way meant to be other than illustrations. Many other questions could be raised and the questions I have raised could be phrased differently. Recognize, therefore, that these questions are only the start of the process in preparing for success with a capitated contract. If the various clauses in the contract are not analyzed and completely understood, and potentially eliminated through questioning once the contract is signed, the provider/group physicians will have to live with that contract. Regardless of the amount of capitation being paid because of the various clauses in the contracts, the physician/providers may still lose money on implementing the contract. Therefore, you will see somewhat of a pattern in the following questions. They are designed to look at the cost of implementing various clauses in the capitated contract. There certainly could be other questions and some are more important than others. So that you can refer back to the actual contract, the questions are in chronological order as they appear in the contract.

1.1.1 The issue of coordination of benefits can affect the bottom line of the physicians/provider group. When physicians sign a contract similar to this, they should know specifically not only who is responsible for collecting appropriate revenues under the coordination of benefit arrangement spelled out in the subscription agreement but also who is going to keep those dollars collected. Usually managed care/capitated contracts refer to other documents such as the various appendices to the contract, amendments to the contract, or in this case, the subscription agreement. Whenever there is such a reference to a document supposedly attached to the contract, those accepting the financial risk for patient care must have a copy of the reported attachment/document and must understand it completely because it is legally binding on the signers of the contract.

1.1.3 This fairly innocuous definition is one potentially costly for the provider. Some managed care companies have spent a lot of time and money to develop an encounter form compatible with their computer system; therefore they want all the providers in their system to use that particular form. On the surface, this is a fairly straightforward and understandable request for the managed care company; remember, however, that many physicians/medical group offices have their own form. If they have to convert to the managed care company's encounter form, there may be a significant cost involved including retraining employees and changing the provider's MIS system. If such changes are anticipated, a question for 1.1.3 would be, who is to pay for any conversion cost to the HMO encounter form?

1.1.5 This section relates to the physician designated by the managed care organization to be the medical director and to perform the duties of the medical director in accordance with the policies of the managed care organization. My question to the managed care company would be about physician/provider input to the selection of the medical director and to the medical director's duties and control over what physicians can do/have to do for patients under the contract. On a related issue, if there is already a medical director, the question might be how was that medical director selected, which criteria were used, and if the contract is being reviewed by primary care physicians what is the specialty of the medical director. If it is different than a primary care physician, will the medical director truly understand the needs, concerns, and patient care activity of the signers of this contract.

1.1.9 This section discusses the per member-per year limitations on referral and hospital charges as established by the managed care company from time to time. This statement raises the issue of how limitations on referrals are set as well as the companion question of what does "from time to time" mean. Certainly the signers of the contract should understand when such clauses are likely to be changed and whether or not they will have any input into that process.

1.1.14 This clause means preferred providers that have been approved by and designated by the managed care company from time to time. Because many physicians already have established referral patterns, they would want to determine in advance who are the current referral providers and what is the approval process for additional preferred providers to be added by the managed care company.

1.1.16 Relates to referral services. This clause raises questions about who will pay for the services of referral physicians. Also, if such services are provided and approved by a preferred provider, does that automatically mean that there has been a discount/capitated arrangement made with that preferred provider?

1.1.20 This clause relates to future potential group and individual contracts between the managed care company and the employer that would obligate the physicians/providers to provide certain services to certain groups of new enrollees. Obviously from a volume standpoint, new contracts are desirable. However, providers should raise the question as to whether there will be any opportunity to review future contracts with new employers if there is any change in the types of services being required under the subscription agreement and whether there is a significant difference between the demographics of the employee group of the new employer as opposed to the demographics of the current patient population under contract. This might be particularly important if a new patient population is coming under a managed care/capitated contract for the first time and there is a strong pent-up demand for medical services in that employee group because previously they had a strong copay/deductible insurance benefit program or no insurance benefit program at all.

3.2 This clause refers to the transfer of patients and the approval of request for such transfers but does not discuss what criteria are used in that approval process. This could affect the physicians/medical group and, therefore, I would question what criteria are used for that approval process.

3.3 This clause pertains to providing services/other products of the managed care company or its affiliates at some point in the future on a discounted fee-for-service basis. The clause then goes on to say that discounted fee-for-service basis is set forth in Appendix E. However, Appendix E contains no fee schedule and only the statement that it will be established from time to time. Obviously anyone responsible for signing such a contract should have looked at Appendix E and found it was deficient and determined through questioning what is the approval process and what are the fee schedules for certain medical and surgical services based on CPT coding.

4.1.2 This contract clause is very important in that it obligates the physicians/medical group to provide certain services based on a 24-hour-a-day basis and potentially to perform some services in the patient's home. It is very important to most providers who are not providing service outside of their own clinic/office or outside of a normal workday to clarify what services are to be provided at what location and at what time during a 24-hour-a-day basis including Saturday and Sunday.

4.2.1 This clause raises several questions. They include why not have the 50 cent PMPM added to the capitation rate and eliminate the medical management fund; if that is not acceptable, be sure to have in writing the reasons why such a fund can be adjusted up or down.

4.2.2 This clause indicates that the physician/medical group must have at least 200 enrollees from the managed care company before they are eligible to participate in the medical management fund and that they should have their practice open to accept new members during a specific period of time. Assuming this goal of 200 is realistic in a given service area, the question to raise is whether the physician/medical group will still be charged the 50 cent PMPM if they have fewer than 200 enrollees from the managed care company.

4.2.3 This clause relating to evaluating the efficiency of participating physicians may or may not be acceptable to potential physicians. Assuming that it is acceptable the question to be raised is whether a quarterly reporting system is sufficient for the participating physicians to know how well they are doing in a given year. Does this provide them enough time to make changes in their practice patterns should such changes be appropriate? Another question would be even if the reports are done on a quarterly basis when are they actually sent to the participating physicians.

4.2.4 This clause relates to the distribution to the physician of funds from the medical management fund. It indicates there will be a distribution if the physician has a favorable variance up to 120 days from the close of the previous accounting period. An obvious question then would be should interest be paid to the physician who has qualified for a payment of the fund from the time period when the managed care organization paid to the physician moneys for achieving goals during a previous time period

4.2.6 This clause, similar to 1.1.1, refers to the coordination of benefits and segregation of recoveries. In this clause, the contract indicates that such moneys recovered will be credited to the medical management fund. Again, it does not indicate who is responsible for collecting those funds; of more importance would be, why should the collected funds go to the medical management funds instead of going directly to the physicians/medical group providing the service.

4.3.1 and 4.3.2 Both of these clauses refer to retroactive adjustments that are basically very beneficial to the managed care company. Remembering this is a capitated contract, note that as soon as an enrollee signs up for a physician/medical group, that provider/organization has legally accepted the financial risk for the medical services to be provided to that new enrollee. Therefore, the managed care company should have the responsibility because of the administrative fee they take out of the premium dollar (usually in the 12 to 18 percent range) to develop appropriate administrative coordination with employers so that the physician/medical group providers immediately receive capitation for the risk they are assuming. Certainly if an enrollee has been receiving care from a provider, and the provider has not been receiving notice from either the employer or the managed care organization that the enrollee/employee is no longer eligible for services, the physician/medical group should not have its capitation retroactively adjusted. However, like all of the clauses in this contract, if this issue is not negotiated out of the contract during the negotiation process, the managed care company has successfully shifted to the provider the risk for services for which the provider was actually not responsible.

5.7 This has a number of points, and each point may affect a physician/medical group differently. However, the fourth point talks about referral physicians accepting payments by the managed care organization as payment in full for covered services. The questions here are who does the negotiating with those referral specialists and if the physician/medical group can negotiate a better contract with some other referral specialists for the same services, can the physicians/medical groups do so.

6.1 This clause refers to inspections but does not talk about when or where inspections can take place and whether or not there is any compensation to the physician/medical group if they have to have employees work overtime in relationship to such inspections.

8.3 This clause refers to high-quality, cost-effective care. These are the most common terms in managed care today. However, the contract does not spell out the policies the physician/medical group must adhere to in providing such high-quality, cost-effective care. The question to raise at this point is does the physician/medical group have the opportunity to review and approve such policies before signing this contract.

9.2 This clause refers to tail coverage and it obligates the physician/medical group providers to provide it. This raises the question as to whether such tail coverage is available and if it is available how expensive will it be to the provider.

11.5 This clause pertains to the managed care company's ability to suspend this agreement. However, nothing in the clause talks about an appeal process when the managed care company decides to suspend the agreement.

I recommend that as part of the negotiating process you ask what is the determining factor to suspend the agreement and what is the appeal process, if any.

Appendix B This breakdown is very appropriate in developing a capitation reimbursement rate for providers. However, in reviewing this you should determine on what basis these rates were set. Be sure they are appropriate to make a comparison between the demographics of the patient population used in determining the rate as compared to the demographics of the patient population of the physician/medical group signing the contract.

Appendix C Lists examples of services covered from the primary physician capitation fund. The heading would lead us to believe that since these are examples, there may be other services not listed here. That would be an obvious question to raise. The other question relates to the fourth point in Appendix C dealing with surgical procedures performed in the physician's office. Such surgical procedures must be spelled out by the CPT-4 code to make sure that the physicians signing this contract are competent and comfortable doing those procedures in their particular offices

Appendix D Appendix D is important but at this point it is nonspecific. You should question what are the guidelines for the development of a service area for the plan obligating the physician/medical group providers specifically either by the number of miles or the number of minutes from the providers' office where services are given to patients.

All of the preceding are but sample questions that can be raised for this particular contract as well as other contracts in the future. This also pertains to the amendment of the contract. Note that capitation rates on schedule one on the amendment (albeit, they may be very appropriate) are different from the capitation rates under the contract from this same managed care organization for potential patients over 65. Again this would raise the question as to what is the appropriate capitation rate based on the current and/or potential patient grouping that the physicians/medical group signers of the contract will have in the future.

Analytical Process for Calculating Capitated/Risk Contract Rates

As physicians and medical groups become more involved with managed care and capitation, they need to be more oriented toward a new businesslike approach to the financial side of their practice. Such a businesslike approach would definitely include knowing what their costs are and having those costs as part of their budgets. Another key part of the budget would be estimating how much revenue is anticipated, particularly under a capitated contract. A budgetary process including an estimate of future managed care/capitated income should be part of an overall, annual strategic and business planning process. As part of that process each year, physicians and medical group leadership or advisors should calculate the potential income and costs of the group, particularly under capitated contracts. As we have indicated earlier, there are various ways to reimburse physicians under capitation. Similarly, there are various ways to develop and calculate capitated contract rates.

As a basis for both contract negotiation and financial planning, you need to identify, define, and calculate some major steps and key philosophical areas so that appropriate financial planning can be made and hopefully implemented effectively. I express my deep appreciation and gratitude to my former colleague,

Madeline Angela Miskowic, now a senior planning analyst for Metropolitan Health Plan, a managed–care subsidiary of Hennepin County Medical Center in Minneapolis for her assistance in developing the following analytical process. I believe that the approach taken by Ms. Miskowic is comprehensive, as well as flexible, depending on the amount of risk to be accepted. It also allows for marketplace differences such as oversupply/undersupply of particular physician specialties and hospital beds. Although this particular model was developed for Minnesota, it certainly can be used as a model and adjusted for different communities in other states. As an introduction to this analytical process, particularly as part of a budgeting process for physicians and medical groups, this process provides a mechanism to evaluate what a provider's approximate cost and capitated payment (PMPM) might be under a capitated contract. We recognize that a number of factors in the contract/negotiation process may change the PMPM payment.

Before a medical group embarks on accepting a capitation contract with a payer, the group should attempt to obtain information on all of the elements that have gone into the budgetary premium PMPM model of that payer. This is important because knowing which elements go into the PMPM premium of the health plan or direct contractor gives the providers more flexibility when they are negotiating their contract. For example, if the health plan is administratively cost effective, are administrative costs kept within 15 percent or less? Is the health plan financially healthy? Does the health plan currently have the sufficient state-required reserves in the bank, usually two or two and one-half months of projected medical costs? If not, will the providers be supplementing the build up of the health plan's reserves, and for how long? Understanding the elements of a capitation premium PMPM model can assist a medical group in asking some of the key questions from Chapters 6–8 that may improve its success in negotiating.

ANALYTICAL PROCESS FOR CALCULATING RISK CONTRACT PMPM RATES

Step 1: Define All Services Included in the Capitation Contract

The first step that a medical group must do with the payer when negotiating a PMPM rate is to define all services included in the capitation contract rate. Also, ask what other variables the third-party payer has included in its PMPM model for premium rate setting for members. Doing this up front gives the group a greater understanding and helps it identify opportunities in the contract negotiation process with the payer.

Although more and more vertically integrated health care delivery systems are coming into existence (e.g., PHOs which in part are developed for the purpose of contracting), medical groups often are approached by payers for individual group practice capitation contracting. If the group wishes to directly contract with a payer and accept a capitated contract rate for medical services only, then the key element of that contract will be to clearly define all medical services the group is to provide or be responsible for in that contract so the group does not take any unplanned or unnecessary risk. In addition, all service exclusions need to be clearly defined in the capitation contract.

Capitation contract rates usually are based on the historical costs and utilization for a particular population of patients. The following formula shows the two essential principles for success or profit in the PMPM ideology. The first principle is that if a medical group can maintain appropriate patient utilization, service frequency may be less than projected. Second, if a medical group can maximize its resources and control costs over 12 months, they can be profitable under an appropriate negotiated capitation arrangement. The formula for calculating a per member per month rate is

PMPM = Service frequency X Average cost/12 months

Often the best scenario in a managed care environment is one in which both the physicians and hospitals are capitated in a mutually beneficial risk contract. Here, if the infrastructure to managed care is in place, physicians and hospitals can maximize care delivery efficiencies and resources for profitability and growth. Usually physicians and hospitals are not willing to take on capitated contract risk arrangements unless the revenue stream from the payer is 15 to 20 percent or more of their total revenues. Whenever physicians and hospitals are working together under the same contract incentives, risk is more manageable. In addition, in this scenario the covered service categories and major cost data are more easily identified because the provider is a comprehensive vertically integrated care delivery system and fewer services will be excluded, thus creating the opportunity for greater control of costs.

> Examples of covered service categories and major cost data necessary to those services include:
>
> ♦ Medical group covered service definitions, prepaid utilization, and charge data.
> ♦ Hospital inpatient covered service definitions, utilization, and charge/cost data.
> ♦ Covered service definitions, utilization, and charge assumptions for referrals to physicians, facilities, and other ancillary services outside of the prepaid medical group.
> ♦ HMO/prepaid plan industry utilization and cost data.
> ♦ Service exclusions.

Step 2: Risk Adjust Medical Services.

A medical group negotiating with a health plan or contractor will need to risk adjust for the specific population of patients it manages under the contract to ensure adequate capitation payments and year-end financial success. The most common risk adjustment performed is the age/sex adjustment. The actuarial chart in Figure 9–1 shows illustrative age/sex adjustment factors. Usually these factors have to be obtained either by an actuarial firm or from the payer. The age ranges and number of males and females in the potential population of patients under contract may potentially be obtained from the payer. The risk-adjustment factor is a relative value index. Generally, the actuarial firm collects service data from multiple third-party payers on various national or regional populations. They may use 4 to 6 million covered lives in their database analysis and include all services related to the populations. A statistical chart of indexes is developed based on age ranges for males and females and how the services fall within the various age/sex categories. Theoretically, if a patient population has a balanced risk, the age/sex

FIGURE 9–1

Actuarial Risk Adjustment Chart

Age Ranges	Male	Female	Composite
0–24	0.597	0.700	0.65
25–34	0.560	1.376	0.99
35–44	0.760	1.209	0.99
45–54	1.287	1.437	1.37
55–64	2.042	1.931	1.99
65+	2.543	2.234	2.39
Total	0.836	1.156	1.00

FIGURE 9–2

PMPM Model for Analyzing Risk Adjusting Medical Services (Payer's proposed composite PMPM rate is $45.)

Age/Sex Category	Payer's Proposed Composite PMPM Rate	Risk Adjustment Factor	Adjusted PMPM Rate	Total Lives	PMPY Total
0–24 (Male)	$45.00	0.597	$26.87	6,890	$6,178.95
25–34	45.00	0.560	25.20	5,733	7,812.00
35–44	45.00	0.750	33.75	21,963	32,602.50
45–54	45.00	1.287	57.92	13,435	174,961.22
55–64	45.00	2.042	91.89	12,451	501,811.29
65+	45.00	2.543	114.44	11,467	3,502,969.79
0–24 (Female)	45.00	0.700	31.50	7,891	9,387.00
25–34	45.00	1.376	61.92	7,342	19,876.32
35–44	45.00	1.209	54.41	22,911	49,562.96
45-54	45.00	1.437	64.67	10,267	79,408.62
55–64	45.00	1.931	86.90	10,833	606,787.79
65+	45.00	2.234	100.53	6,746	678,175.38
Total				57,086	$5,669,533.80
Divide Total Number of Lives into Total Revenues					$99.32
Divide PMPY by 12 Months to Obtain PMPM					$8.28
Multiply Frequency by PMPM* 5.6885					$47.08

*Frequency of service may come from historical data service for the particular population being cared for by the physician. It may come directly from the third-party payer, or it may be actuarial in nature, which is a composite of many covered lives often specific to a geographic region.

risk indicator would equal one. An increase in risk equals more than one and a decrease in risk equals less than one. This composite age/sex index can be used to multiply against either utilization to obtain target utilization for a given population of patients. It can also be used to adjust revenues for a specific population.

The medical group can use the actuarial age/sex data, which is based on national statistics of very large patient populations and applies to all specialties, to compare/analyze their PMPM proposed rate from the contractor (see Figure 9–2).

Step 3: Identify All Other Variables Included in the PMPM Premium Rate Model of the Health Plan or Direct Contractor.

Undoubtedly, the biggest percentage of the PMPM goes into pre-paid medical services. However, other variables affect the total PMPM rate (see the Comprehensive PMPM Capitation Model). These variables include:

- All prepaid medical services (as previously described).
- (Add) Other outside referral costs not included in the PMPM.
- (Less) Copayment revenue.
- (Add) Reinsurance premium.
- (Less) Reinsurance recoveries.
- (Less) Interest income if applicable.
- (Add) State reserves (generally 2 percent of total).
- (Less) Coordination of benefits.
- (Add) Premium tax, if applicable.
- (Add) Profit.

Step 4: Adjust for current HMO/Health Plan Demographic Factors (for example, premium community rating structures).

At the end of the comprehensive PMPM capitation model is an HMO/Health plan adjustment factor. This factor is generally a composite of various key indexes used by health plans to adjust their premium rates. The following steps reflect how those individual indexes may be developed and

FIGURE 9-3

Year 1 Premium Adjustment by Quarters

1st Quarter	$162.00	=	(11 X $160 + 1 X $184)/12
2nd Quarter	$168.00	=	(8 X $160 + 4 X $184)/12
3rd Quarter	$174.00	=	(5 X $160 + 7 X $184)/12
4th Quarter	$180.00	=	(2 X $160 + 10 X $184)/12

Year 1 = $160 PMPM Year 2 = $184 PMPM (CPI increase of 15%)

used. To simplify this discussion, a composite index was developed from the individual indexes described later. For example, the HMO demographic factor is 0.9919 in the PMPM capitation model. HMO indexes may include:

1.   **Inflation factors:** A quarterly premium rate adjustment is usually done by the health plan so that the targeted revenue PMPM can be achieved each month and the plan remains solvent. These adjustments usually are based on various specific published medical CPIs (Consumer Price Index) or the all medical CPI. The health plan may or may not adjust premium rates and provider capitation rates based on their quarterly results/CPI until year-end or the next open enrollment period. Examples of quarterly premium adjustments are in Figure 9–3.

2.   **Premium rate structures and rates:** Now that the Health Plan premium rates have been determined, the health plan then calculates a single rate conversion factor (CF) to adjust the set premium rate. Before it can do this, the plan must identify the premium rating structures it will use; these include

♦ Single rate composite structure   Employee
                                                            (includingall eligible
                                                            dependents)

♦ Two-tier rate structure*   Employee only
                                                            Employee and one or
                                                            more dependents

♦ Three-tier rate structure*   Employee only

*Most frequently used.

	Employee and one dependent
	Employee and two or more dependents
♦ Four-tier rate structure	Employee only
	Employee and spouse
	Employee and dependent children
	Employee and spouse and dependent children
♦ Four-tier (Alternate)	Employee only
	Employee and one dependent
	Employee and two or three dependents
	Employee and four or more dependents

As shown, there are a variety of premium rating structures. Providers need to be aware of the two key underlying principles which govern how rates may be set by a health plan. These two key factors may affect the success of the health plan and their contracted providers. First, premium rates should reasonably reflect the approximate total costs by contract type. This ensures that the premium revenue will cover medical expenses and the health plan remains solvent. Second, premium rates should be reasonably *competitive* with the marketplace to ensure maintaining market share.

The formula for developing a premium rate for each tier rating structure is

Three-Tier	Number of Persons per	Ratio to

$$1. \text{ Capitation Rate} = \frac{\text{Avg. Premium per Contract}}{\text{Avg. Members per Contract}} = \frac{\text{Average Premium}}{\text{per Member}}$$

To calculate unknown single premium rate CF to adjust premium rates, the formula is

2. Capitation Rate X $\dfrac{\text{Avg. Contract Size}}{\text{Avg. Premium Units}}$ = Conversion Factor (CF) for a Single Rate (S)

Premium Rate	Contracts	Contract	
Single	40%	1	1
Two persons	20	2	2
Family	40	4.1	3

Conversion Factor = $\dfrac{0.40 \times 1 + 0.20 \times 2 + 0.40 \times 4.1}{0.40 \times 1 + 0.20 \times 2 + 0.40 \times 3}$

= $\dfrac{2.44}{2.00}$ = 1.220

Capitation (Year 1—1st Quarter) = $161.31 (from capitation PMPM model)

Example: if S (single rate) = 1.22 (CF) for a three-tier premium rating structure, the adjusted rates might be the following recognizing that for market share/competition reasons the actual rates could go up or down.

Single premium (S) rate	= $161.31 X 1.22	= $196.80
Two-person premium rate	= $196.80 X 2	= $393.60
Family premium rate	= $196.80 X 3	= $590.40

3.   **Community rating flexibility:** The reality of the competitive local marketplace may inhibit the health plan from charging its members simple community-rated premiums as just described. Therefore, additional factors are taken into consideration. These factors include a variety of options allowed under current federal law giving the health plans flexible rating mechanisms. Some state laws, particularly over the last two years of the state health care

FIGURE 9-4

Comprehensive PMPM Capitation Model for Total Risk

Hospital Services	Utilization	Avg. Chg	Gross Cost PMPM	Copay	Copay PMPM	Cost PMPM	C.O.B.	Net Cost PMPM
Inpatient	0.25	$1,783.58	$37.31	$50	$1.05	$36.26	–$0.87	$35.39
Extended care	0.01	403.62	0.34			0.34		0.34
Same day surgery	0.05	1,221.96	5.19			5.19	–$0.08	5.11
E.R. PAR	0.26	121.79	2.62	$25	0.54	2.08		2.08
E.R. NON PAR	0.01	470.98	0.51	$50	0.05	0.46		0.46
Other	0.35	230.87	6.73			6.73	–0.06	6.67
Subtotal			52.7		1.64	51.06	–1.01	50.05
Primary Care								
PCP cost	2.38	116.7	23.12	$5	0.99	21.48		21.48
Subtotal			23.12		0.99	21.48		21.48
Physician Services								
Office visits	0.6	62.5	3.11			3.11		3.11
Periodic exams	0.01	67.49	0.05			0.05		0.05
Inpatient visits	0.1	115.15	0.94			0.94		0.94
E.R. visits	0.17	114.79	1.62			1.62		1.62
Misc. office svcs.	0.16	13.58	0.18			0.18		0.18
Surgery								
Inpatient	0.07	872.32	5.31			5.31	–0.04	5.27
Same Day	0.11	412.83	3.92			3.92	–0.02	3.9
Assistant	0.01	767.6	0.51			0.51		0.51
Anesthesia	0.04	753.47	2.7			2.7	–0.01	2.69
Maternity	0.01	5,462.84	5.96			5.96	–0.03	5.93

Service	Freq	Avg Charge	Gross PMPM	Copay	Copay PMPM	Net PMPM	Adjustment	Adj Net PMPM
Mental health/chem. dep.								
Inpatient	0.01	131.97	0.05		0.05			0.05
Outpatient	0.77	67.83	4.34	$5	0.32	4.02		4.02
Alcoholism								
Inpatient	0.01	76.07	0.03		0.01	0.03		0.03
Outpatient	0	147.02	0.02	$54		0.01		0.01
Laboratory	1.32	13.41	1.47			1.47		1.47
X-ray	0.43	68.74	2.49			2.49		2.49
Therapy	0.21	51.15						
Other	2.82	63.21	14.88			14.88	-0.06	14.82
Subtotal			47.57		0.33	47.24	-0.16	47.08
Other Services								
Prosthetics/DME	0	64.75	0.01			0.01		0.01
Ambulance	0.12	63.79	0.62			0.62		0.62
Home health	0.25	84.86	1.75	$5.00		1.64		1.64
Infertility	0.01	177.05	0.1		0.1	0.1		0.1
Other	0	141.09	0			0		0
Subtotal			2.47		0.1	2.37		2.37
Net total			$125.86		$3.06	$122.15	-$1.17	$120.98

Administrative overhead (12% of premium) — $19.36

Reinsurance (6% of premium) — $9.68

State reserve (2% of premium) — $3.23

Other admin, mkting, debt service, premium tax, and Profit (5% of premium) — $8.07 — $40.33

*Total Cost PMPM — $161.31 — $160.00

Adjustment for current HMO demographic Factor = 0.9919

*Freq × Avg. Charge/12 mo = PMPM

Source: **Madeline Angela Miskowic**, 1995, Minneapolis

reform movements, prohibit the use of some of these federally approved rating systems. Federally approved rating mechanisms include:

♦ Geographic indexes or governmental units. Indexes for city, school district, state employees, and other experience ratings reflect an individual community or population.

♦ Administrative and market expense flexibility rate setting by group size. Federal regulations allow premium variations for groups of less than 100 subscribers or groups of 100 and more subscribers.

♦ Realignment of rates to match in-force rates for federally qualified HMOs. The ratio of rates can be varied to match the in-force indemnity insurance rates in a given community.

♦ Rates can be varied by contract distribution and family size.

♦ Family rates can be varied to reflect different dependent eligibility definitions for enrolled groups.

♦ The ratio between family and single rates may be adjusted to reflect more accurately the cost relationship between two contract types.

♦ Community rating by class. This rating method classifies all health plan members into classes actuarially derived or based on certain factors that predict differences in utilization of HMO services by individuals or families in each class. Our age/sex risk adjustment factor is a simplified version of this methodology.

Final Adjusted PMPM Capitation Model

Composite Community Rating Factors	Derived Index
Single premium (S) rate	1.2200
Geographic index	0.8000
Administrative market index	0.9530
Adjustment for current HMO demographic factor, composite rating	0.9919

♦ Experience rating: Some states have prohibited experience rating under their current health care (reform) legislation. In experience rating, group members might be assigned to one of three or more classes. Those classes might be defined as:

FIGURE 9–5

Capitation Payment Distribution Model

	$160 PMPM premium	
	$40.33 (-$0.91)= $39.42 HMO Marketing/ Administration	
$50.05 Hospital	$21.48 PCPs	$47.08 Physician network/ risk-bearing entity

Class One: A community-rated class includes all employer groups of between 25 and 100.

Class Two: Fully experience-rated class includes all groups between 500 and 1,000 employees.

Class Three: Groups of more than 1,000 generally have their premiums based on a weighted average of their own experience and the community rating by class rates for the group.

Figure 9–5 illustrates the distribution of the premium dollars of the PMPM capitation model. Actual distribution may vary significantly based on contract negotiation, the composition of and structure of the physicians and/or hospitals being capitated, as well as the needs of the specific patient population being cared for under the contract.

KEY MANAGED CARE PERFORMANCE INDICATORS

The preceding analytical steps help in defining the key performance indicators monitored under the capitation contract. The key performance indicators vary depending on the physician mix, the level of services, and the level of integration under the capitation contract. A comprehensive model of key indicators may look like Figure 9–6.

FIGURE 9–6

Key Managed Care Performance Indicators for a Comprehensive PHO
(HMO XYZ Capitation Contract) (YTD December 31, 1994)

Membership			Financial		
Membership	57,086		Total revenue		
Member months	465,822		Actual		$78,944,255
Market share	28%		PMPM		169.47
			Budgeted		85,000,000
			PMPM		182.47
			Variance		(6,055,745)
Inpatient Care			Percent variance		-7.12%
Admissions	5,635				
Admissions/1,000	145				
			Total expenses		
			Actual		$75,069,020
Patient days	20,445		PMPM		161.15
Patient days/1,000	539		Budgeted		82,875,000
			PMPM		177.91
			Variance		(7,805,980)
ALOS	3.63		Percent variance		-9.42%
Newborns	1,695				
per 1,000 F. Ages 10–49	45				
			Surplus		
			Actual		$3,875,235
			PMPM		8.32
Ambulatory Care			Budgeted		2,125,000
ER visits	12,762		PMPM		4.56
ER visits/1,000	329		Variance		1,750,235
			Percent variance		54.84%
			Surplus margin		-4.91%
Outpatient enc.	119,075				
Rate/member/year	3.07				
			Health expenses		
			Actual		$63,808,667
Laboratory claims	149,464		PMPM		136.98
Rate/member/year	3.85				
			Administrative expenses		
			Actual		$11,260,353
Radiology claims	19,924		Percent of revenue		14.26%
Rate/member/year	0.93		PMPM		$24.17
Pharmacy $ PMPM	$16.40				

Admits/1,000 = Admits/member months *12*1000
ALOS = Average length of stay
PMPM= Total $/total member months

ABC Clinic Emergency Room Utilization Incentive Monitoring

*Admits/1,000 = Admits/member months*12*1000
*ALOS = Average length of stay
*PMPM = Total $/total member months

1994

HMO XYZ	QTR 1	QTR 2	QTR 3	QTR 4	Total
ER visits	3,090	3,191	3,255	3,226	12,762
Member months	116,450	114,962	118,211	116,199	465,822
ER visits per 1,000	325	320	304	365	329
Projected ER visits assuming no change					
year end 1993 for 1994: Visits/1,000					14,120
Difference between actual and projected					1,358
Multiplied by $40 incentive payment per visit under 1994 projected utilization:					$40
1994 Incentive payment based on comparison of year-end 1993 data					$54,320

PROVIDER INCENTIVES AND REWARDS

Finally, capitation contracts should reward their providers for appropriate utilization and efficient resource management. This is usually done through provider incentive programs, often written into the contracts. For example, one of the most controversial and targeted performance monitorings is emergency room utilization. If a provider group is able to manage ER visits well, then the difference between the actual ER visit rate and the projected PMPM ER visit rate on which the PMPM contract is based, might be paid to the medical group in a contract bonus. The above example is an ER utilization incentive monitoring model.

The number of elements represented in the payer's PMPM capitation model suggests that health plans have significant flexibility in setting member premium rates, as well as proposed provider capitation rates. Medical groups who understand the health plan premium rate setting process, as well as risk/rewards, have a competitive advantage in negotiating their contract rates and risk arrangements. They are not only able to see more clearly the opportunities and pitfalls in the proposed contract arrangements but also recognize the need to implement the contract clauses in a cost effective manner to have a profit at year-end.

10

How to Develop a Managed Care Strategy:
Remember You Only Get What You Negotiate

Much has been written and said about the process of negotiating managed care contracts and particularly capitated contracts. As an example, it is relatively easy to say that the best negotiating posture in managed care negotiations is to negotiate from a position of strength. Unfortunately, for the majority of physicians and their administrators who are not experienced with managed care contracts and negotiating, it's the other side that usually has the strength. Normally, the managed care organization has a team of experienced negotiators/lawyers who understand the financial and legal implications of the contract they want physicians to sign. Depending on the financial implications of the contract (i.e., over $100,000 versus only thousands of dollars), the managed care organization will probably have three people representing their organization at the negotiation sessions. Those three are likely to include someone from management, someone from the MCO's financial department, and someone who represents the legal/contract department of the MCO, possibly an attorney. In such an environment how can physicians and medical groups possibly negotiate from strength? By developing a managed care strategy.

The starting point for most physician practices/medical groups in developing a managed care strategy is to define their contracting objectives to fit with their group's mission statement and goals. Obviously if the physician practice/medical group has never developed a mission statement/strategic plan the time to do so is before getting into managed care contracts. During the process of defining the provider's own objectives in a managed care environment, the providers can look toward and compare a particular managed care organization's objectives. Depending on the competition and marketing in a given service area, and the openness of the managed care organization's management, such a comparison may be achievable in varied degrees.

PRACTICE STRATEGIC ANALYSIS

To assist providers with the development of a managed care strategy, and in defining their managed care objectives, I recommend that providers develop a *practice strategic analysis.*

The strategic analysis uses as its base the information the providers/medical group gained by going through their practice activity analysis as outlined in Chapter 6. The potential of negotiating from strength requires the providers to have as much information about the patient base as does the managed care company. Because the managed care company is already getting a great deal of information from other providers, particularly hospitals, it is important when approaching a new managed care contract that the providers/medical group understand not only as much about their own practice but also how that practice fits with comparative costs of providing care in that medical service area. To do that the providers need to know which of their services are costing the most for managed care organizations, particularly acute, inpatient care. Therefore, the provider/medical group should determine what the other physicians, potentially the competition, are doing with the local hospital/hospitals as far as admissions by specialty/physician, length of stay, procedures, and services provided to those patients as well as the average charges/cost for those patients. Hopefully, a part of the physicians/ group managed care strategy would be to develop information from the strategic analysis indicating that your particular practice/medical group are more cost effective providers for the services in your service area than your competition. Particularly as you get into capitation where reimbursement rates often are based on best average cost in the medical service area, it is a valuable help in negotiating to know your own costs prior to being offered a capitation rate based on average community costs.

Speaking of reimbursement, part of the strategic analysis should be a comparison of reimbursement from different managed care organizations for the same services. As we indicated earlier, different managed care models also have various methods of reimbursement. Assuming that some patients may shift between managed care organizations, part of your strategic analysis should be to determine the impact on your bottom line if you have the same patients but a different reimbursement from a different managed care organization. At the same time you should recognize that the costs of doing business under one managed care organization may be more or less than the company you are currently negotiating with. At this point, it becomes extremely important to go back to the information from Chapter 6 and take a look at your own demographic data. Hopefully this includes an employer/third-party payer mix, and if so, do a trending analysis of what is happening with your current patient load.

Gathering and understanding the impact on your practice of demographic information may help you develop a negotiating strategy. Such information helps you determine what unique features your practice/medical group has, particularly in comparison to other comparable providers. Such unique features might include the location or locations of your practice/medical group. In addition to the convenience/attractiveness of parking at given locations, as part of your negotiation strategy, you need patient satisfaction survey results. These surveys should come from not only patients but also potential patients and employers in the service areas near each practice location. This may cost some money but it will often provide, in writing, a negotiation strength that may assist providers in either getting a higher reimbursement rate or a contract over their competitors. Such surveys would certainly include the availability and value of special services/procedures which, like an ambulatory surgical center, may have cost effective value to the managed care organization.

Also, strategic analysis assessment should include a statement about the value of the name recognition of the provider practice/medical group/organization. Managed care companies trying to expand their market penetration, in particular, are much more likely to negotiate a favorable contract with a provider practice/medical group that already has a strong patient base and quality name recognition, as compared to a new organization that has just started.

At this point in your strategic analysis it will be very helpful to determine the alternatives your patients have compared to receiving care from your organization/the managed care organization. This should include the cost of receiving that care and where such patients will receive specialty care if hospitalization is necessary.

To best use the information you have pulled together in your strategic analysis, combine this information with your current cost structure and patient services utilization, for each physician in the practice. Many physician practices do a very good job of understanding what their charges are to their patients for various services, usually by CPT–4 codes. Some practices and medical groups track this information and have an understanding of reimbursement by various payors of those same services. These are particularly valuable parts of the pricing strategy that you need to develop as part of your overall managed care strategy. Unfortunately, many practices and group/network/physician organizations don't know their actual costs of providing those services, particularly by CPT–4 code. As we discuss in Chapter 14, it is particularly important to have an understanding of the cost of your services by the CPT–4 codes, and then to figure out the appropriate use of that information. Basically you want to at least know the CPT–4 codes that produce 80 percent of the revenue for the practice. This will help you decide what you want to provide or not provide under managed care reimbursement.

FINANCIAL RISK ASSESSMENT

The next part of your managed care strategy is often determined by the types of managed care contracts being offered to providers in the community either from managed care companies or from direct contracting with employers and coalitions. Specifically before signing a managed care contract each provider organization needs to do its own internal *financial risk assessment* for different types of contracts. As we pointed out earlier, most physician practices today are still professional corporations used to distributing their available cash on December 31, to avoid unnecessary taxation. Therefore they have little, if any, in the way of cash reserves. Particularly, for these medical practices, the financial risk assessment is very important. The actuarial aspects of a reimbursement rate, particularly a capitated rate, in a managed care contract will have included in it a potential for some percentage of high-cost patients, as well as low-cost patients. The shifting of financial risk from third-party payers to the providers can be handled in various ways such as the development of risk corridors and/or stop loss insurance. However, the strategy in dealing with the managed care organization is to determine what are appropriate risk corridors and/or how much stop loss insurance may or may not be necessary as part of a contract. This can only be done rationally if the providers have developed a financial risk assessment, based on their current and projected financial situation.

Particularly in relation to the financial risk assessment, but also as part of the overall managed care strategy, is the need to assess the providers' service utilization. If the physicians in a given practice/medical group are on a productivity income distribution system, whereby the tests and services they order result in a higher amount of income distributed to that particular physician, the service utilization by physician/service code is very important. In such situations, particularly if the managed care contract is going to have reimbursement based on the provider/medical group doing/improving their utilization review activities, an assessment on almost a physician by physician basis is necessary to determine if the utilization patterns will change, or could be changed, depending on the contract's financial incentives particularly under capitation. In Chapter 12 on income distribution under capitation, we discuss in greater detail the need for aligning financial incentives for individual physicians with the type of managed care contracts which are signed.

COUNTERPROPOSAL PREPARATION

At this point, the providers/medical groups should have gathered a great deal of information to be used in the development of a negotiation strategy for the proposed contract as part of the group's managed care strategy. Assuming the provider/medical group has received a contract from a managed care organization for the provider's consideration, now is the time to take the information gathered and to develop a counterproposal. Obviously managed care organizations are very pleased when providers sign the contract as presented to them without any discussion or changes being negotiated. In reality the providers should want to negotiate a number of changes as part of the contract process. Therefore, this is the time to develop a counterproposal to assist the provider/medical group in making the decisions it needs to make to justify signing the proposed contract.

As part of the counterproposal strategy, physicians/groups need to develop a financial model of the impact of the contract as proposed by the MCO and compare it with a financial model/models that reflect the changes the providers want to have made in the contract as part of their counterproposal. Obviously the financial modeling needs to include a variety of factors generated by the strategic analysis, as well as by the analysis of the proposed contract itself. Note that often times one of the most important models that should be developed is one that shows the result if the providers do not accept the contract from this particular managed care organization at all. Obviously such a model should include the potential of a volume shift of patients away from the practice and the resulting costs of either restructuring the practice or the changes that may be created by a drop in the practice revenue/physician's individual income. Without doing some financial modeling, providers may accept a managed care contract and end up basically discounting either some fee-for-service rates or accepting some other contract rate at a deeper discount for services to patients that the provider/medical group is already serving.

Another strategy approach would be the possible concern that too much of the practice's volume is with one managed care organization. When possible, even if it will cause some decrease in per patient revenue in the short run, it may be advantageous to long-term financial survival to add another competing managed care organization contract to the providers' total third-party payers. As we have previously stated, there is no one best answer to each managed care contract proposed to providers. It is only through the development of a managed care strategy and strategic analysis procedures that sound business decisions can be made for the future benefit of the practice. These sound decisions need to be coordinated into a negotiation strategy that has specific goals and minimum fallback positions already made before entering into actual negotiations.

As the providers and their negotiation team approach the actual negotiations, it is best to start from the standpoint of understanding the strengths and weaknesses of the managed care organization. Recognizing that the MCO usually negotiates in teams, it is then best for the provider organization to have a similar team. This should include a specific spokesperson, so identified, as well as someone on the team who will be taking notes of what both sides say. A provider organization that does not have a great deal of experience with such contract negotiations should hire experienced consultants and legal advisors to assist with negotiations. Such advisors should be familiar with the types of contracts being offered and the financial ramifications of the various clauses that are part of those contracts.

Assuming that as part of their negotiating teams both sides bring to the negotiation table individuals who can accept or decline offers during any part of the negotiation process, it is usually most advisable to not be too quick to accept an offer or to change a particular part of the contract. Throughout the process, remain fixed on your strategy and plan for future changes in the contract. During the process, the possible changes negotiated usually should be taken back and worked through a new financial model prior to final decision making. At this point the physician/medical group should have a better understanding of this very important process. Because of the future financial impact of this process on all providers, it is worth emphasizing, *you only get what you negotiate. And remember, you'll get more the more prepared you are for each stage of the contract process.*

11

CHAPTER

Recognizing the Change and Impact of Going from Discounted Fee-for-Service Contracts to Capitation

It would be easy to simply indicate that physicians needed to be aware that under capitation the financial risk for the cost of care of a given patient population has been shifted from the third-party payer to the physician or the physician's medical group. The basic assumption in most parts of the United States is that when physicians and medical groups enter into capitated contracts, they are at risk for losing money because of the lower capitation rate. However, physicians and medical group leaders/advisors should recognize that capitated contracts can be financially very rewarding. The financial reward depends on the group's capability and negotiating skills in achieving a reasonable capitation rate; equally important is to agree to a contract that is implemented with minimal additional cost. My experience is that implementation of the contract, depending on the specifics of various contract clauses, can be as beneficial or as costly to the physician/medical group as successful rate negotiation for the contract.

We have already talked about the various aspects of a contract. Note that there are differences in the way that capitation

FIGURE 11–1

Capitation Dollar Flow Example

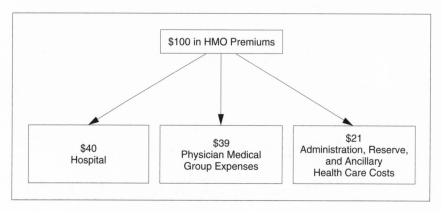

can be structured and how these changes impact the amount of financial risk for the physician/medical group. One of the keys to successful capitated contracting relates to who is accepting the full risk for patients and how that full risk is subdivided among primary care and specialty physicians. Figure 11–1 shows how capitation dollars flow. This simplified model indicates that from the $100 premium, $40 goes to hospital costs, $39 goes to physician/medical group expenses, and $21 is withheld for administrative costs and other expenses including reserves and marketing.

The inclusion of the hospital usually is desired by the third-party payor, particularly when acute inpatient care is covered by the contract. A hospital that is going to accept financial risk under capitation wants to partner with the physician/medical groups who actually control the amount of services provided patients in the hospital setting. Therefore, it becomes fairly obvious when total health care costs are negotiated in the capitated contract that the success of that contract for the providers would normally require the hospital and physician/medical groups to have the same incentives in the implementation of that particular contract. Most third-party payors believe that when the incentives for all providers, including the hospitals in the system are in alignment, the total costs for patients within the system will be controlled with a result that will be beneficial to the third-party payor by the end of the year. How the hospital and physicians/medical groups actually implement that contract, even if their incentives are aligned, determines the financial success of the contract at the end of the term.

As indicated earlier, the philosophical and financial change for most providers under capitation is that they have now accepted financial risk. Certainly depending on the experiences of the providers with capitation, it is vitally important that a sufficient number of patients be covered under the contract. This is assuming these patients have their medical care in essence prepaid by the third-party payor on a per member per month (PMPM) capitated rate to the providers. Managed care actuaries, who are key to understanding and determining appropriate capitated rates, indicate there is safety in numbers. For example, a small primary care group that starts a capitated contract by assuming full risk for its patients and not having at least several thousand enrollees under that contract, runs the statistical risk of a major financial disaster at any point in the contract year. To continue the example, if the primary care group was willing to accept full responsibility for the total care of a given population of 200 patients, and the capitation rate was $100/month for each of these 200 patients, there would be a steady cash flow of $20,000 per month. From a statistical standpoint, the providers in this illustration may think a percentage of these patients won't even need care during the contract period and therefore they can be fairly comfortable since the contract produces $240,000 in total for the group during the year. However, the statistical outliers may easily diminish that $240,000 cash flow into a negative financial position even before the end of the year. Certainly with primary care physicians there may be patients enrolled in their population of 200 who might have children born during that contract period. Should one of those births become premature twins, requiring four to five weeks in the neonatal intensive care nursery of the hospital, the entire year's cash flow may disappear with that one family's birth expenses.

These types of horror stories are sometimes real and sometimes exaggerated. The reason that they are sometimes exaggerated is that in many cases a capitated contract can be negotiated that will allow the provider to buy as part of the contract stop loss insurance that covers the financial risk for a patient over a certain dollar amount in a given contract. This stop loss insurance, depending on who the third-party payer is, can often be arranged by reducing the amount of capitation paid to the providers each month to cover the cost of the stop loss insurance. The key for controlling the financial risk is: First, have a viable number of enrollees under the capitated contract. This number should be in the vicinity of 5,000 to 10,000 enrollees. Second, even with a statistically adequate number of enrollees such as 10,000, each individual provider/medical group needs to determine how much financial risk it thinks it wants to accept. Some experienced groups may want to accept the entire financial risk, even with less than 5,000 enrollees under a particular contract. Others may always want to be on the conservative side and have stop loss insurance that would kick in at $20,000 or $40,000 of cost per enrollee per year. Obviously the trade-off between the $20,000 or the $40,000 per year per stop loss insurance per enrollee is how much would be deducted from the capitation rate paid monthly to the provider.

Earlier we mentioned the wide spectrum of capitated contracts. Such contracts include subcapitation of specialists by an organization (i.e., an integrated delivery system) that has accepted full risk from the third-party payer. The subcapitation is used in a carve out arrangement so that the integrated delivery system will be subcontracting on a capitated basis with specialists like radiology and anesthesiology. Sometimes the integrated delivery system may accept a full risk capitated contract and then subcontract with physicians/medical groups on a modified fee-for-service contractual arrangement.

Often times the arrangements for subcontracting depend on the availability and capability of the primary care physicians to act as gatekeepers. When there are gatekeepers (i.e., primary care physicians), the patients will normally either request or be assigned to a specific primary care physician. Following the assignment of the patient to a given primary care physician, that physician, acting as a gatekeeper, usually controls the access of those patients to specialists and inpatient acute care. With some capitated contracts the gatekeepers can subcontract to specific given specialists for their patients. In other circumstances, the patients can go to a wide variety of specialists who are part of the integrated delivery system's total panel of physicians providing service to patients under that given contract. The situation varies from city to city but where there is an integrated delivery system accepting a full contract from a third party-payer, the integrated delivery system institutes economic credentialing to have only cost-effective providers on their panel.

The 1980s a saw strong drive toward developing independent physician associations (IPAs) as a way for physicians to participate in the managed care contracting process. Usually the development of IPAs included trying to have as many physicians as possible sign up for the panel of providers in those IPAs. Under capitation, besides the financial risk that physicians may have in accepting capitated reimbursement, physicians need to be aware of their economic credentialing. The big question and difference from IPAs is whether physicians meet the criteria that the third-party payors or the integrated delivery systems are looking for. If not, physicians may not find themselves on the list of physicians that patients under that particular contract can go to for care. Certainly with an oversupply of some medical specialties today, albeit in the larger cities and metropolitan areas, the trend in the 1990s is to direct patients to specific physicians who have been evaluated and approved through an economic credentialing process. As the managed care environment has become more and more competitive, the move to only include cost-effective providers is growing as part of the strategy of the successful MCO, particularly in the capitated environment.

Certainly most providers moving into the capitated contract arena need to focus on the capitation rate as it pertains to the particular patient population. Obviously a well-informed actuary with managed care experience can be very helpful in assisting providers with statistical approaches to a given patient population. We all understand that 200 female patients of childbearing age are much more likely to have higher medical costs than 200 males 30 to 40 years old. Therefore, in considering a capitated contract, efforts must be made to determine the demographics of the total potential patient population by age and gender. Such information is very helpful to the actuaries in giving some statistical probabilities to the occurrence of the outliers who may need more expensive inpatient acute care such as

FIGURE 11–2

Example of Decreasing Revenue from Increased HMO Volume

Scenario I
HMO Market Share
30%

	HMO Members	FFS Patients	Total
Population	720,000	1,680,000	2,400,000
Number of procedures	70,000	252,000	322,220
Number of patients	46,800	168,000	214,800
Revenue at avg. chg.	$33,345,000	$119,700,000	$153,045,000
Percent rev. HMO vs. FFS	21.79%	78.21%	

Scenario II
HMO Market Share
55%

	HMO Members	FFS Patients	Total	Compare
Population	1,320,000	1,080,000	2,400,000	
Number of Procedures	128,700	162,000	290,000	-9.78%
Revenue of Patients	85,800	108,000	193,800	-9.78%
Revenue at avg.chg.	61,132,500	$76,950,000	$138,082,500	-9.78%
Percent rev. HMO vs. FFS	44.27%	55.73%		

Assumptions for example only:		Utilization (weight average)	
Average charge/procedure	$475.00	HMO/1000 (example)	65
Population	2,400,000	FFS/1000 (example)	100
		Number of procedures/patient	1.5

coronary artery bypass surgery. Additionally, different work populations may have a tendency toward more costly expenses. For example, the employees in the postal department may lift a lot of boxes and sacks of mail; this could create more orthopedic problems than computer programmers working at computers. Such a potentially adverse patient mix needs to be carefully considered in negotiating total capitated fee reimbursement rates.

We need to reemphasize the importance of alignment of financial incentives for all involved with a capitated contract. Looking at Figure 11–2, note the two scenarios on it indicating the impact when the percentage of managed care/HMO market activity increases from 30 percent in scenario 1 to 55 percent in scenario 2. The resulting changes for the number of patients, the number of procedures, and the revenue per average charge by going from 30 to 55 percent, drops approximately 9.78 percent. Although it does not necessarily have to be that way, if we assume that all of this change is related to more capitation as a form of reimbursement, it becomes very obvious that the reduction of procedures and revenue will impact all providers, including the hospitals in the system participating in the contract. Therefore, all providers who are impacted by a capitated contract should be aware that there needs to be a cooperative, risk-sharing approach to the signing and implementation of capitated contracts. Obviously the approach of all involved in the implementation of the capitated contract will change from previous discounted fee-for-service contract in that a bed in the hospital may be more valuable empty than if it is filled. Remember that under capitation all services and patient utilization become costs for the signers of the contract since the capitated income is paid to those same providers based on the number of enrollees under contract by a per member per month (PMPM) reimbursement, not on the volume of service provided.

The critical distinction then under a full capitation contract is that the provider's income also depends on the effective case management and health education of all of the patients/employees covered under that particular contract. Usually the focus changes to be more on preventative and primary care designed to help reduce total system expense, while at the same time allowing for a profit at the end of the contract for all of the at risk providers. Chapter 12 addresses the importance of physicians in a medical group realigning their financial incentives for their income distribution system as their medical group accepts capitated contracts and a larger and larger share of their total revenue from capitation.

Physicians/medical groups going into negotiation and then implementation of their first capitated contract must recognize that they are going through a transition process. Equally important is recognizing that the contract itself has a time frame of one year, two years, or three years after which the contract will be renegotiated, assuming that the experience has been at least somewhat beneficial for all of the providers who accepted the financial risk of that contract. Several other chapters toward the end of this book are devoted to issues and activities to assist physicians in medical groups with the implementation of their capitated contracts (i.e., cost accounting and computer systems). During the transition, which would include the planning for making the decision to accept a capitated contract as well as the actual negotiation and then starting implementation of the contract, physicians and their medical group leadership should keep in mind that this process to capitation can have either a positive financial upside or dangerously negative downside. Therefore, we recommend that physicians and medical group leadership become well informed about the ins and outs of capitated contracting and the impact of capitated contracts on physician practices.

Hopefully, you already realize that it is usually very helpful to get assistance from experienced advisors who have been through capitation wars on more than one occasion. Certainly the legal issues involved in the contract, which we cover in Chapter 15, should require advice from a health care attorney who understands the impact of the various clauses of the contract from an operational and financial standpoint and not just the legal standpoint. Some physicians in medical groups recognize that they do not have the expertise to protect themselves in this type of contract activity. Therefore they turn to consultants or management service organizations (MSOs) that can provide the assistance necessary in both the contract negotiation stage and the implementation stage, so that the physicians/medical group can have a positive financial outcome from the capitated contract. When physicians/medical groups enter into capitated contracts as part of an integrated delivery service total contract, they need to anticipate that there will be MCO networkwide or delivery system protocols relating to patient utilization and quality performance standards. In contracts this may sound relatively innocuous. However, in implementation the burden of developing or adhering to networkwide protocols can be frustrating, time consuming, and costly. Also there is a difference in the way that physicians and patients interact under capitation.

Many integrated delivery systems with capitated contracts spend a lot of time and money on patient health education, on new telephone triage systems, on availability of substitute non-ER services (i.e. urgent care centers), and the development of grievance procedures so that patients who feel they are not being treated satisfactorily can complain to someone other than their physicians. Often these complaints are not necessarily related to physician care. Instead they are related to the rules and regulations imposed on the patient by the system or plan that in some patients' minds equate with a lack of appropriate care. Growing out of the importance of providing a new educational approach to patients, such changes produce change not only for the physicians new to a capitated system but also their nurses and other personnel who assist physicians in the patient's care. This is particularly true in competitive marketplaces where marketing competition between various capitated plans often uses patient satisfaction surveys as a mechanism to evaluate physicians and their support staff. Assuming positive results of the survey, competitors then market to new or potential enrollees that the physicians and employees of plan A provide much better service than the physicians and support staff of plan B.

Although many other potential areas considered in the transition to capitation may not be universal for all providers, one last major thought about transition is particularly important for physician specialists and subspecialists and the leadership of their group practices. This last thought is that the basic underlying approach in capitation shifts the focus, and often the capital, to primary care providers. Often times the primary care providers under these contracts are called the gatekeepers. The shift of focus for hospitals, the specialists, and the subspecialists must be recognized as the gatekeepers now develop and exercise a great deal more influence over the total care of and costs from capitated patients, including their referral to hospitals and specialists. Particularly under an integrated delivery system approach to a fully capitated contract, responsibility for the financial success for the total contract shifts to the primary care physicians. Therefore, all providers and their support staffs who provide care within the system under the capitated contract must work with and assist the primary care physicians in successfully developing protocols and utilization management approaches to cost-effective, quality care.

Recognizing that some of the previous information is a radical change from the good old fee-for-service days, I close this chapter by reminding you of two things: The first is that readers of this book five years from now will be somewhat amused because this book is designed for physicians and medical groups moving into capitation from the fee-for-service reimbursement arena. They will be amused because most physicians and medical groups within five years will have converted to some form of capitation including totally capitated patient populations with no fee-for-service. The second reminder comes from Marilou M. King, Esq., Executive Vice President, National Health Lawyers Association, who said in April 1994, "the survivors in the twentyfirst century would be those integrated systems with a comprehensive array of clinical services who had learned how to accept risk under capitation."

Physician Income Distribution Systems under Capitation

Previously we have discussed the importance of coordinating financial incentives for providers in the managed care environment. Certainly this is most true and necessary when the reimbursement from managed care is in the form of capitation. When discussing the alignment of financial incentives, it is assumed that the providers include the hospital/hospitals as well as physicians/medical groups and other providers who are all participating in a full risk contract. However, this chapter discusses the importance of appropriate incentives for the physicians, particularly those with medical groups that currently have the more traditional productivity type of income distribution systems. There is a very important need to have the physician income distribution system change its alignment of incentives so that all of the impacted physicians are more concerned about the new total bottom line of the group from capitation, as opposed to the traditional productivity of the group as measured by more and more gross dollar volume. Under most managed care systems, the emphasis is based on cost containment strategies. We see the income distribution systems of physician groups moving to the same type of strategy when they find that a significant proportion of their total dollar volume is being generated from managed care contracts, particularly capitated contracts.

As one of three consultants who surveyed and analyzed the results of more than 20,000 physicians in 250 medical groups in the 1994 Survey of Physician Income and Productivity for the American Group Practice Association, I am well aware of the changing trends from physician/medical groups across the country in their medical income distribution systems. Traditionally many single specialty and smaller medical groups have been on a production-based income distribution system. The basis for such a widespread system was the predominance of fee-for-service as the main type of reimbursement for physician services in the 1960s and 1970s. As some markets became more involved with managed care in the 1980s and 1990s, the compensation plans for physicians started to shift from 100 percent production plans like salary plus incentives, salary plus production credits, and, in some cases, straight salaries for physicians in larger multispecialty group practices. In some single specialty practices, where the partners previously agree to basically all share equally, that philosophy under managed care shifts somewhat to where all physicians basically receive a salary. The results of that very large survey for the American Group Practice Association showed that nearly 33 percent of the groups with less than 35 physicians based their physician compensation solely on production, while only 19 percent of the groups with more than 100 physicians paid solely on production. When there was a combination of salary and production, the production proportion ranged from 10 to 95 percent. In groups with more than 100 physicians, over 81 percent have a component of salary and 67 percent are based primarily on salary. This is in contrast to the smallest groups where 66 percent have a salary component and 45 percent are primarily salary.

That survey also found that more than 23 percent of the physician groups indicated they were planning to make a change in their compensation system within a year. *Nearly all of the groups contemplating changes planned to move toward systems based on less production and more salary or salary plus incentives.* Remember that in 1994 when the survey was completed, there was a concern among physician groups relating not only to managed care and capitation reimbursement but also to the changes in federal legislation which were pertinent to physician's income distribution systems as discussed in the Stark II bill. Legislation passed by Congress in 1994 indicated that physician/medical group's income distribution systems starting January 1, 1995, needed to be tested against the new regulations of the Stark II provisions. The incentive compensation design in a distribution formula needed to become aware and adhere to the restrictions set forth in the legislation 1877(H)(4)(a)(iv) that basically indicated physicians who are members of a group practice may not receive compensation on the volume or value of referrals. That legislation did indicate physicians in a group practice, however, could be paid a share of overall profits of the group or a productivity bonus based on services personally performed or services incident to such personally performed services, so long as the share or bonus is not determined in any manner directly related to the volume or value of referrals.

Obviously with managed care and capitation growing rapidly across the country, with the state and federal governments moving Medicaid and Medicare patients into managed care programs, and with the Stark II legislation, physicians and medical groups have felt the need to change their income distribution systems. In addition, physicians, medical group leadership, and their financial advisors have learned that production-based income distribution systems do not work well under capitation. A capitation distribution system based solely on production is not logical because capitation has an inverted relationship to the old fee-for-service production philosophy. On the other end of the scale, capitation income distribution formulas that are basically 100 percent salary do not allow for credits such as for individual physician cost effectiveness/performance and overall contribution to their medical group.

In 1994, Jon Lewis, Angie Miskowic, and I developed a new model income distribution system for physician groups receiving most or all of their revenue from capitation.[1] We designed the new model as a guide and format for appropriate incentives in an income distribution system under capitation because under capitation the medical group and its physician are at financial risk. Obviously each group of physicians approaching the challenge of changing their income distribution systems needs to take into consideration a number of similar issues and then develop

---

[1] John F. McCally, Jon Lewis, and Angie Misckowic. "Capitation Income Distribution Systems: They're Better with a New Approach," *AGP Journal*, September/October 1994, pp. 48–50, 52.

FIGURE 12-1

Income Distribution Model for Medical Group's Capitated Reimbursement

Example: A group of 10 MDs, a single specialty group, and an example of one of those physicians who has been with the group for nine years.

Group's distributable income for physician compensation (DIPC), estimated after paying expenses: $2,000,000

I. Base salary—25% (2,000,000 x 25%) = $500,000.
    Dr. X = $500,000 divided by 10 = $50,000

II. Seniority factor—5% of DIPC
    Seniority split (5% X $2,000,000) = $100,000
    Seniority calculated by internal point system based on number of years' service.

Dr. X 9/140 points x $100,000 = $6,428.57

(Note: 140 is the total number of seniority years for all 10 physicians.)

III. Production credits—50% ($2,000,000 X 50%) = $1,000,000
     Dr. X's production credits: (Maximum allowable is 2 points of each 5 production categories or 10% of total points for this pool.)

Cost per patient credit	1.5
Utilization credit	1.0
Fee-for-service equivalent credit (pts>35 per day)	1.0
Patient service credit	0.0
Case management credit	1.5

Dr. X's total production credits = 5 points = 0.083 of total production credits X $1,000,000 = $83,000

(Total points available for all doctors was 60 points)

IV. Performance credits—15% ($2,000,000 X 15%) = $300,000
    (Maximum allowable is 2 points of each of the 5 performance categories or 10% of total points for this pool)

Dr. X's Performance Credits:	
Continuing education credit	1.0
Board certified through 2 boards	1.0
General contributions to group	1.5
Administrative duties to group	0.5
Overall performance contribution	1.5

Dr. X's total performance credits = 5.5 points = 0.092 x $300,000 = $27,500

(Total points available for all doctors was 60 points)

Figure 12-1 (concluded)

V. At risk withhold for extra costs/possible bonuses—5%
    Money held back this accounting period (usually calendar year) for next year:
    (5% X $2,000,000) = $100,000. Funds for distribution from last accounting
    period: $50,000 includes interest earned. As approved by the board of
    directors: Equal split for good team cost effectiveness in: (1) patient encounters;
    (2) appropriate number of referrals;(3) appropriate amount of lab, X-ray, and Rx.

Dr. X's Bonus Income $50,000 divided by 10 M.D.s = $5,000

Summary of Dr. X's Total Income:

Base Salary	$ 50,000.00
Seniority	$ 6,428.57
Production	$ 83,000.00
Performance	$ 27,500.00
Bonus	$ 5,000.00
Dr. X's total income	**$171,928.57**

Source: John McCally, Jon Lewis, and Angie Miskowic, "Capitation Income Distribution Systems: They're Better with a New Approach," *AGP Journal*, September/October 1994, pp. 48–50, 52.

specifics based on what is happening in their marketplace, with their specific managed care contracts and particularly capitated reimbursement. The model in Figure 12–1 model is one which allows for flexibility in the design of a new system, particularly for those physicians in medical groups making the transition from fee-for-service to capitated income.

Under a capitated managed care contract, a provider/medical group enters into an arrangement with the payer, to share or accept the risk of providing some or all medical services to a defined population of enrollees/employees. This risk sharing, potentially constant revenue, and variable patient costs are the reasons behind the necessity for developing an equitable physician income distribution system for capitated reimbursement that provides appropriate physician incentives. As such, a new, well-designed income distribution system should reward those providers who provide both cost-effective and high-quality care.

There is no good cookie-cutter method for developing new income distribution systems, particularly for capitated reimbursement. However, my colleagues and I believe five major factors are important to include when creating a new formula or redesigning a group's current income distribution formula to handle capitation successfully. In Figure 12–1, we have designed a hypothetical model using five major factors for a group of 10 physicians in a single specialty, and using $2 million of distributable income. Figure 12–2 illustrates the percentages of using the same five factors for distributing compensation to a group of physicians. The leadership/partners of each group will want to approve/assign their own weights to each of the five major factors and various subfactors depending on the group's size, past history/income distribution methods, and future projections of managed care/capitated income.

1. **Base salary**—up to 25 percent of each physician's total compensation may be shared income based on his/her medical specialty, taking into consideration competitive national, state, and even regional compensation norms. Fringe benefit allowances may be considered; that is, the amount of benefit expenses to be paid by the group for each physician.

2. **Seniority**—up to 5 percent of the total dollars available for distribution may be allocated using points for each year of physician tenure as a partner.

3. **Production credits**—up to 50 percent may include a cost per patient (CPP) credit. This is done through comparative analysis of CPP within the practice or within the community with credits for the following categories.

> *Utilization credits* may be considered for capitated income. This generally refers to a physician's referral patterns within and outside the group.
>
> Some groups may use a fee-for-service equivalent credit that can prevent penalizing the physician with high volume and difficult caseloads.
>
> Another production credit may be a *patient service credit*. This comes in the form of actual quality assurance/patient satisfaction surveys. Some clinics have patient survey questionnaires that patients fill out when they leave.
>
> Another credit that can be given is *case management credit*. This credit is given for good patient case management from start to finish of care. This type

of credit is likely to be more common in the future under managed care programs and mandatory outcomes data reporting requirements.

Finally, credits may be given for appropriate *prescription drug management.*

4. **Performance incentives**—can be weighted up to 15 percent. They are used as a tool to motivate, evaluate, and commend a physician's contribution to the practice/group. Examples of these credits would be:

   Continuing medical education credit.

   Board certification credit.

   General contributions to the group.

   Updating and improving medical or operational procedures.

   Administrative contribution credit for those who take on leadership or medical operational duties (i.e., medical director).

   Overall performance credit.

5. **At risk compensation**—can be up to 5 percent of the total available income pool, withheld from distribution for at least one accounting period (one year) and given as bonuses when group objectives have been attained. Group objectives may include patient encounter targets met, referral targets met, appropriate use of the number of lab and X-ray tests performed, and overall financial objectives being met.

My colleagues and I believe that the preceding formula provides a rational and equitable approach to distributing capitated income. Because every medical group is unique in its physician/specialty distribution, patient volume, managed care contracts, and financial goals/growth, the factors and percentages in Figure 12–2 can be modified to fit any group.

My colleagues and I strongly recommend developing a new income distribution system under capitation. Such an approach should include a major communications program to ensure physician participation and understanding before the system is implemented. This is particularly true when a medical group is making a transition from a total fee-for-service based production plan to a capitated income distribution system.

FIGURE 12–2

Capitation (income distribution model)

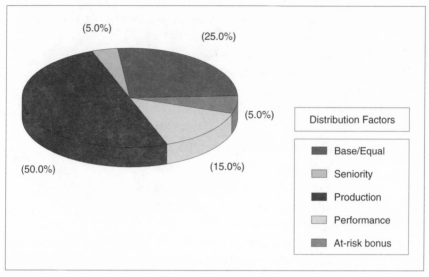

Source: John F. McCally,Jon Lewis and Angie Miskowic, "Capitation Income Distribution Systems: They're Better with a New Approach," *APG Journal*, September/October 1994, pp. 48–50, 52.

Because of the wide variety of factors affecting each medical group, there is no one right way of designing a distribution system for capitated reimbursement. However, the wrong way is to not have adequate controls/incentives in the distribution formula to prevent over-utilization and to not allow rewards for quality care and cost efficiency.

As previously mentioned, one of the key reasons for changing income distribution formulas under capitation is that the medical group has usually accepted financial risk when negotiating a capitated contract. Our model income distribution system could assist physicians in the planning and implementation of the capitated contract to avoid any adverse financial risk. A number of other areas in each contract also help in averting an adverse financial situation from happening under capitation. Certainly the need for cost accounting and management information systems as outlined in following chapters is a part of the necessary implementation of a capitated contract to avoid the potential downside risk. Unless all of the physicians in the group have and follow appropriate incentives to be cost effective providers, however, they will not be successful in the future as a group under capitation. We believe that our model for income distribution systems under capitation helps significantly to provide for all the physicians in a group to have similar incentives to successfully implement the capitated contract.

DISTRIBUTING CAPITATED INCOME IN SMALL PRACTICES

Changes from capitated revenue can easily impact even two physicians practicing together. As we become more aware that under capitation the focus needs to be on financial risk and costs, it becomes more important to have the physicians sharing similar financial incentives. Historically, under fee-for-service and productivity-based income distribution systems, this was not difficult. Under capitation there are more options, however, and it is more difficult to get accurate financial information related to the costs of a practice and the RBRVS production. As you can see from the following examples, there are multiple ways to approach distributing the capitated revenue of a practice. As with the transition to any new income distribution system, to be successful will likely require an investment of time and resources to create the right system for your practice.

Example 1: Distribution model of capitated income based on productivity percentages

This is the scenario for both examples:

Primary care physician's income pool is $150 per patient per year × 3000 patients for two MDs; that is, $12.50 PMPM (per patient per month) which equals a total patient revenue of $450,000 from HMO XYZ. In this model, we assume both physicians could have traditional non-HMO patients also.

Production	MD 1	MD 2	Totals
HMO gross production (based on fee-for-service billing)	$285,000 (45%)	$345,000 (55%)	$630,000
CAPITATION			

Hold 40% of capitated revenue for overhead and at risk pool/investments = <-$180,000>

$450,000 − $180,000 = $270,000

Available income for distribution for two MDs = $270,000

Distribution	MD 1	MD 2
Using traditional productivity percentages approach	$270,000 X 45% = $121,500	$270,000 X 55% = $148,500

Example 2: Distribution model of capitated physician income based on RBRVS and UR costs

Cost-Based Production	MD 1	MD 2	Total
HMO production based on RBRVS and/or HMO reimbursement levels	$202,500	$247,500	$450,000
Medical service cost per patient ($/pt/yr) (based on estimated internal UR costs and external referral expenses)	$75,000 (37%) ($50/pt/yr)	$105,000 (42%) ($70/pt/yr)	$180,000

Available capitated income
for distribution:$450,000 (Total Capitation) – $180,000 (Costs) = $270,000

Distribution of revenue available for physicians based on production costs	$127,500 ($202,500- 75,000)	$142,500 ($247,500- 105,000)	$270,000

Other options for distributing the $270,000 available between the physicians:

		MD 1	MD 2
1.	A 50/50 split of available capitated revenue	$135,000	$135,000
2.	A year-end cost containment credit to the 50/50 split based on which doctor is more cost effective	37% $141,750	42% $128,250

MD 1 is paid 5 percent more than MD 2 from the equal split of capitated funds available for distribution.

Other possibilities for credits in allocating income may include:

♦ Recognition of intangible/nonquantifiable contributions.

♦ Recognizing quality of care.

♦ Recognizing overall performance and contributions to the practice such as utilization and efficiency.

13

CHAPTER

Management Information Systems Improve the Chances for Success of a Capitated Contract

Timely, appropriate information is the key to success in implementing a managed care contract. Many physicians/medical groups' computer systems and software deal with the accounts receivable activities for physicians and their patients. Under capitation, where the cash flow for each capitated patient does not depend on the amount of services provided to a patient, nor the efficiency in billing and collecting for those services, there is a major need for looking at other aspects of the physician's practice activities; for example, their costs and related capitated revenue. In many offices, this cannot be achieved with current medical group software billing systems that focus on accounts receivable. Capitation usually does not result until physicians and medical groups have become integrated to the point where they can accept risk and capitated contracts; remember that appropriate information is crucial for determining the success of that integration, often clinically as well as financially. As we discuss in the next chapter on cost accounting, it is very important to have an appropriate information system for physicians/medical groups to compare actual experience against expectations.

Those expectations need to be part of a flexible budgeting process with variance reporting. Normally this type of information system capability is not available with the more traditional MIS systems used in many physician offices/group practices today. Certainly as we saw in earlier chapters, profit under capitated reimbursement is created as the end product of the capitated revenues received, minus the costs for the services associated with providing services to capitated patients. Additionally, since President Clinton's proposed Health Security Act of 1993, there will be a continued emphasis on patient outcomes from those services. Technically, this requires a linking of the financial information related to the patient's care with the outcomes of that care. Then there will be the need to have an interaction electronically between both the cost/revenue information and the patient's outcomes data with the management information system necessary to monitor and manage the capitated contract itself.

The process of capitated contracting is more than just the negotiating of the initial contract. The success of implementing that capitated contract depends on the ability of the management information system to provide appropriate feedback information to the physicians/medical group management. They need to compare expectations against actual activity and then do appropriate modeling and forecasting, including what-if analysis relating to the financial and activity trends being developed for the patient care provided under a capitated contract. I have advised my physician/medical group clients in the past that when they enter into a capitated contract it should be with the thought that this is not a one-time event. Rather it should be the start of a continuing, successful relationship between a provider organization and a third-party payor. For that relationship to be successful, the provider organization must be able to track, trend, and make projections with and through their own management information systems. This is particularly true at the end of the contract year when the contract is being renegotiated. At this point the management information system is a very necessary tool in providing timely, appropriate data for the decision-making process and for renegotiating the contract for the future.

When used as a tool for renegotiating the contract, the management information system (MIS) looks at a number of key factors as part of the modeling and what-if analysis process. Those key factors definitely include the volume of patients, particularly those capitated at the start of the contract year, as well as those added or dropped during the year and those that are anticipated being added in the future by the managed care company in its marketing efforts to third-party payors. Another key factor obviously relates to the capitation payment itself. However, the capitated rate itself is only partially helpful in the modeling because profit under capitation comes from the need to be able to subtract from the capitated revenue the associated cost for providing services for that group of capitated patients. Obviously to do that, the provider's management information system needs to track and project services from a cost standpoint and not just from the capitated revenue standpoint. This is particularly true if the capitation includes inpatient services that are usually much more expensive than ambulatory services. Further management information service modeling should definitely include inpatient/specialty care if included in the capitation rate, particularly the lengths of stay by diagnostic service codes provided by each of the physicians in the group. Other key factors to be included would be the tracking of risk sharing provisions, particularly outlier clauses in the contract, and the financial impact on the group/providers of service to certain outlier patients, which may create the largest portion of costs associated with the capitated contract.

All of these issues are part of the management reporting activity necessary for successful implementing and monitoring of capitated contracting by physicians/medical groups. This management reporting, using a good management information system, helps the provider/decision makers focus on both the incremental and long-term impacts developing from their decision to accept and implement a capitated contract. Those incremental impacts focus on financial issues raised in the last paragraph, as well as several other key areas. The first of those is the ongoing utilization review activity of the provider/medical group. This is particularly important when there are multiple physicians in a group who previously had not participated in utilization review programs.

Second, depending on the type of contract and the range of services covered by the contract, the physicians/medical group leadership must be track through its MIS referral authorizations and IBNRs. Many physicians can understand and have a good idea as to how they personally can control the cost of patient care under capitalization. However, particularly if it is a primary care group referring patients for services to specialists, there needs to be a tracking mechanism for monitoring both the approval, at an appropriate service level, and the subsequent cost to the original provider group of services by the referral specialists who take care of referred patients. Incurred But Not Reported (IBNRs) are costs which sometimes do not even get billed by the end of the contract year, much less paid, to the original physician/medical group responsible for the cost of the care under the capitated contract. Particularly the IBNRs for expensive services, such as coronary artery bypass surgery, need to be tracked not only from the cost standpoint but also from the standpoint of monitoring the outcomes of services by other physician providers not capitated by the contract.

Third, the physician provider group must monitor the enrollee population covered by the capitated contract. Employees leave and/or are hired by employers every month. Different employers have different arrangements, but basically within 90 days new employees have the opportunity to sign up for a specific benefit program/health care provider or once a year employees are offered the opportunity to switch benefit plans/providers. Under capitation, as soon as the employee has signed up for a given provider/medical group, that provider/medical group immediately becomes at risk for the care of that patient. Therefore, the physician/medical group must have a MIS that keeps track of employees who have signed up for their services. Providers need to determine for every patient their eligibility for care and, on a monthly basis, what is the appropriate amount of capitated revenue that the provider/medical group should be receiving for those eligible enrollees. Similarly, as employees leave the employer and are no longer entitled to the health care benefits, the provider's management information system must be informed appropriately so that it does not provide services for which the provider/medical group is not receiving capitation at that point. Management information systems, therefore, need to keep current on enrollee status, and to monitor appropriate payments for enrollee status; often this can be done best by electronic interchange of information between the provider and either the managed care company or the employer directly.

Some physicians/medical groups that sign capitated contracts look to the HMO/managed care company to provide them with the previous information. Remember, however, that with more than 500 HMOs and 1,000 PPOs, there is a wide spectrum of capabilities with managed care organizations as to the timing and usefulness of information from their management information systems. Particularly rapidly growing HMOs and PPOs have had difficulty keeping current with their internal management information systems. On the other hand, most managed care organizations recognize the importance of having appropriate, accurate, and updated management information systems.

As an example, I quote Dr. William W. McGuire, the president of United Healthcare, one of the nation's largest investor-owned, managed care companies. He said, "We need to achieve desired clinical outcomes at appropriate costs." And the way to achieve that goal he said, "is by influencing people with information." He went on to say, "if we are going to succeed, we have to change behavior" and "the best way to change behavior is to gather more information, analyze it in meaningful ways and share it with others." Note that United Healthcare has already gained national publicity by publishing report cards that offer consumers information on the performance of various of its health plans. Because United Healthcare has been in business for many years, it has had the opportunity to develop sophisticated management information systems. Particularly during the negotiation and renegotiation stages of capitated contracting with managed care organizations like United Healthcare, be aware that the managed care organization usually has a much better, more sophisticated MIS and database. However, even with sophisticated companies such as United Healthcare, which is one of the nation's largest managed care companies with plans in more than 25 states, their focus is to continue expansion of health care automation in the years to come. Dr. McGuire commented, "the EDI [electronic data interchange] highway is going to have a vast range of capabilities, ranging from traditional claims management to the profiling of clinical practices. This will result in the reengineering of the health care delivery system."

Obviously, this chapter represents a significant change from the good old days when there were no computers in physicians' offices or if there were, they were used only for billing and collections. Today management information systems for managed care are management tools for providing considerable data including a detailed analysis of a provider's financial performance under managed care contracts. Such performance should include the utilization patterns of providers as discussed earlier; when coupled with the modeling MIS also allows for the development of appropriate managed care strategies and sometimes, specific managed care strategies for individual managed care contracts. All of this points out again that most health care providers today are part of multimillion dollar businesses. And, as with most multimillion dollar businesses, they need to expect that part of the cost of doing business will be the acquisition and use of appropriate managed care management information systems. These continue to improve and become more sophisticated. As such, the computers providers buy today will not be the same ones they will be using five years from today. Between now and then there will be increased integration with clinical core data, marketing information, and other external systems on a real-time basis. Certainly the ability to bring together both financial and quality of care information will be critical to managed care companies and physicians/medical group providers in the future.

Speaking of the future, providers/medical groups will have more and more interface with employers and the agencies of the federal and state government who pay for health care. Certainly both employers and the federal and state agencies dealing with the physicians/medical groups will be very concerned about the providers' ability to be cost effective and manage their enrollees' care so there will be quality outcomes. To do that, utilization and cost data will be extremely important. As an example, some employers/third-party payors will want to determine whether the care from a specific provider/medical group provides higher-quality outcomes and/or more cost-effective care than from a different set of providers/medical groups. Such comparisons, particularly with the oversupply of certain physician specialties, make it imperative for physicians and medical groups today to develop, analyze, and produce information that will be as positive as possible regarding the care provided by that particular provider organization. Such information truly can be developed only by appropriate management information systems.

Speaking of employers, there may arise competing interests for the database information which providers have on employees of those employers/third-party payers. The ownership and control of information, including the analysis of that information relating to multiple parties, can be a very complex and controversial issue. Thus, the managed care/capitated contract must spell out in detail the agreement between the employers, the managed care organizations, and the providers as to the control of medical and financial data, as well as the rights and interests of employees/patients concerning privacy and confidentiality. Because the health care delivery system is now market driven, there is no way of predicting where the future needs of management information systems will stop for providers. What is very apparent is the need for physicians/medical groups to actively be prepared and working on developing better and more cost-effective management information systems for the future.

The Benefits of Using Cost Information When Implementing Capitated Contracts

We have introduced several cost accounting terms previously in this book when we looked at the chart of capitation showing fixed costs and variable costs equaling total costs. When those total costs exceed the provider's fixed capitated revenue, the provider experiences a loss rather than profit. Today many providers don't know which of their costs are related to implementing health care services, particularly under a capitated contract. This chapter can help physicians/administrators recognize the benefits of cost management systems, particularly as they relate to implementing capitated contracts and being able to tell in real time whether they are profiting from capitated contracts.

Previously I had discussed the importance of having timely and appropriate information when analyzing contracts, for developing financial models to determine the impact of potential contracts, and certainly for developing managed care strategic plans, including strategic plans for dealing with a particular contract. What types of appropriate information do physicians and their administrators need to have, and understand, to do these things successfully?

Physician groups moving into capitation and still retaining a portion of their practice and patient mix from fee-for-service and discounted fee-for-service managed care plans particularly need the ability to allocate and trace certain costs of providing different types of patient services to specific cost centers.

Usually within specific cost centers there is a need to separate cost into the fixed components versus the variable components of costs. This is particularly true under a capitated contract where the profit is made for the group/providers by keeping the total costs as low as possible and definitely lower than the amount of capitation received in a particular time segment. The activities involved with such cost allocations are important not only when trying to determine the financial viability of a capitated contract but also as medical groups get larger; truly the financial aspects of these million dollar businesses, including the cost of operations, must be measured and understood. This includes monitoring on a monthly basis the progress or lack of progress as measured against financial projections and an annual budget. Such budgeting in health care delivery today for physicians/medical groups includes the evaluation by physicians/administrators of the impact of their patient volume, case mix, labor skill/cost levels, and variable costs relating to specific contracts and certain cost centers. Having worked with physicians on financial issues since the end of the 1950s, I know that most physicians do not want to spend a lot of time on this subject. So, I have endeavored to make the remainder of this chapter as helpful, yet as nontechnical, as possible. This chapter also relates to the benefit of understanding and applying what is covered in Chapter 10, the successful implementation of the physician's capitated contract.

Because this chapter is designed to prepare physicians/medical groups for implementing capitated contracts, remember that a great deal of time and effort needs to be spent in understanding the financial activities/cost of those services required by contracts. Those services may be considered reimbursable to the physician on a monthly basis in the form of PMPM capitation but don't generate actual costs until there is a patient-physician contact. This chapter primarily highlights key cost management terminology/practices particularly as they relate to capitation.

There are a number of approaches to allocating costs in most businesses. The first of at least two areas identified within the physician/medical group practice is the traditional cost center. The cost centers in the typical physician/medical group practice do not provide medical services to patients but are important to the overall ability of physicians to care for their patients. A good example might be the areas devoted to the storage and control of the patients' medical records; these are necessary for the physicians to use when patients are there for care or as a reference when patients call the physician or nurse for advice on refilling a prescription. Other typical cost centers would include the parking facility, a reception area, and office space for administration. The cost involved with these areas can be measured and then compared on an actual versus budgeted basis, as well as compared to similar costs in other medical facilities. Particularly as a physician/medical group practice becomes more capitated, the goal is to minimize the dollars of expense per unit of activity in each of the identified cost centers for that organization.

The next key area is the medical service activity center. As the name would imply, these are areas where patients receive a type of medical service. These activity areas therefore would have not only expense associated with them but also revenue. Under a capitated contract, the revenue is basically determined by the number of patients assigned to that particular activity center (usually a medical practice specialty area—family practice, pediatrics, internal medicine, OB/gyn), and the expenses for that activity center would be those related to the services provided to patients seen in that activity center. In an overly simplistic approach, the fixed costs which are part of the cost centers of the organization, are determined and assigned in an allocation process to the activity centers. Such fixed costs may be assignable on a square footage basis or on a per unit basis related to activity such as patient visits or patients assigned to a given activity center. When those fixed costs are added to the variable costs allocated to this specific activity center, such as medical supplies, a combined /total cost can then be used as a measurement against the activity center revenue generated by PMPM capitation.

Once such a simple accounting approach has been developed, it can be used for budget variance analysis, as well as the income

distribution systems designed for rewarding physicians who understand and implement cost effective service to capitated patients.
This also becomes very helpful in developing annual budgets and
financial models for analyzing new capitated contracts, or capitated
contracts about to be renewed.

Although it would seem like a relatively straightforward
process, the difficulty with the approach just outlined is that there
are many variables and different interpretations by different individuals within an organization as to what costs should be allocated
and in what percentage to what activity. Books have been written
on cost accounting to help educate those individuals working full
time with the cost side of a business. For the purposes of this book,
and initial clarity, I describe a relatively simple and straightforward
process that can be enhanced as the practice grows and the amount
of capitated revenue increases. The first step in a decision-making
process by the physician leadership/administration of a medical
group starts with the identification of the activity centers to be
measured. This could be as simple as each individual physician, or
as previously mentioned, all physicians within each specialty. A
word of warning: as physicians/medical groups are trying to work
through this process for the first time, they may first identify the
activity centers only tentatively until the rest of the following
process is completed.

The second step in the process is to determine the fixed costs
for the entire organization and how the different types of fixed
costs will be allocated; that is, occupancy costs may be based on
square footage, whereas medical records cost may be based on the
cost per patient for each medical record.

Third, there is a need to identify the variable costs for each of
the activity centers. This in itself can be a time-consuming process
as some costs are not entirely chargeable to one activity center. For
example, the phone receptionist or appointment scheduler may be
providing services for multiple activity centers and therefore such
costs need to be allocated on a percentage basis.

The fourth step in the process may be relatively easy if all
patients are capitated or somewhat difficult if there is a mix of
capitated and other types of patients. This step is to capture all of
the revenues generated by a particular activity center. This
would include obviously the allocation to a particular activity

center of appropriate revenue (after expenses) generated by laboratory services. Recall that such allocation currently needs to conform with the Stark-II federal regulations. I say currently as many state and federal regulations keep changing, particularly as they are administered by agencies such as HCFA or interpreted by the courts. Again, if the activity center's patients are all capitated, the determination of revenue by that activity center is relatively straightforward; that is, the amount of capitation PMPM for the enrollees in the plan assigned to the physicians in that particular activity center.

The fifth step in implementing a cost system for capitation is to actually identify the cost of various services provided in the activity centers. This may include developing a methodology for the allocation of a physician's salary/benefits to each of the services provided by that physician. Recognize that under capitation, this allocation of the individual's expense might become very skewed if the patients who are assigned to a given physician are relatively healthy in a given time period, (i.e., one month), and the physician needs to provide only a limited amount of service during that time. Additionally, the cost of providing service in other activity centers, such as allocating costs to the services provided in a laboratory, need to be determined and allocated to each revenue-producing activity. Now you can bring together fixed and variable costs within each activity center and make comparisons to the revenues generated by that activity center. Once combined, you can use this information as the basis for good fiscal budgeting.

As we have said earlier, the capitated contract will definitely change the physician/medical group's approach to budgeting. In developing the capitated budget, it is important to gather and analyze historical data which we assume was not generated by capitated contracts. The analysis of that data can point out seasonal trends and other variables/activities for patient encounters and procedures performed; such an analysis can be the basis for comparisons with services under the capitated contract.

The collection of the historical data also becomes important when analyzing the managed care organization's data that it used for developing the proposed capitation rate. Certainly physicians/medical groups going into capitation for the first time need to carefully analyze their own practice patterns and patient mix to determine whether the proposed capitation rate was based on similar data and is comparable/appropriate for the physician/medical group. A comparison of the services to be provided under the capitated contract also needs to be made with the physician/medical group's historical data; for example, if the practice previously had been doing EKGs and there is no reimbursement for EKGs during the contract period then the analysis of the data would bring about a different conclusion. Based on the contract, the budget for revenue can be estimated and then traced on a monthly basis. Such information/comparisons can also be used during the renegotiation process to determine whether or not the now estimated revenue does cover all of the costs now being identified under a cost management system.

The preceding outline of a cost management system for capitation is an illustration on a very simplistic basis. It does not include how to account for IBNRs, capital expenditures, depreciation, nor the development of cash reserves. These items and many more are part of the ongoing process of developing appropriate financial approaches to handling capitated contract revenues and costs, as well as running your practice as a multimillion dollar business. The Medical Group Management Association and some consulting firms have a number of valid and appropriate resources that can be used in taking the concept of a capitated cost management system much further into the development of a total accounting and cost management system for the physician practice/medical group of the future.

CHAPTER

Legal Concerns and Issues in the Managed Care/Capitated Health Care Delivery System

Federal and state governments are moving more and more patients into managed care programs. At the same time, they are developing more and more regulations and legislation dealing with the new forms of practice being created by physicians/medical groups/hospitals/PHOs/integrated delivery systems and foundations. In the past antitrust issues have been of concern to physicians, hospitals, and managed care organizations that tried to develop new formats and organizations in the more competitive managed care marketplaces. Recently we have had Stark-II legislation controlling how physicians/medical groups' income distribution systems can treat ancillary service revenue. In addition to the many laws and regulations affecting physicians and the way they practice today, many state laws affect and control managed care companies and the way they deliver care through physicians/medical groups. While this chapter highlights some key legal issues relating to physicians/medical groups in the managed care environment, it by no means answers all legal questions or substitutes for getting experienced and competent managed care and legal advice when necessary.

State governments regulate the practice of insurance and usually the assumption of risk by a company when health care services are provided to a specific patient population for a specific reimbursement. In the past, the insurance companies and HMOs often assumed that financial risk. Today we also have integrated delivery systems of various providers that have come together and have negotiated risk contracts, as well as some physician networks and physician medical groups that provide services to defined patient populations and are at risk for their care. At any given time, there are states that may all be moving in the same direction of regulating providers who are taking risks, or just some states on other health care delivery issues like "any willing provider" regulations. In reality, the implementation of new laws and the new regulation of old laws for managed care companies and providers varies considerably from state to state depending on a number of factors. Some of the differences between states can be explained by how much political clout insurance/managed care companies have or the influence of a state medical/hospital association in a given state. In most states that have passed new regulations for providers assuming risk, those state requirements usually pertain to the providers being able to prove solvency and appropriate financial reserves. Some states have a requirement that the provider organization needs to file with the state insurance department a bond for a sizable sum. For example, $1 or $2 million would be used by the state in case of insolvency or other failure of the provider organization (at-risk organizations) to provide the services from contracts approved by the state. As part of the licensing and approval process of managed care/providers assuming risk, in addition to financial reserves many states require the provider organization to prove it can provide the necessary services for the planned patient population through its provider/network arrangements.

The whole issue of state regulations and licensing of health care providers gets more complicated when there is a relationship between providers and a self-insured employer organization providing employee benefits through ERISA (Employee Retirement Income Security Act of 1974). Usually employers that provide health benefits to employees under a self-insured plan find their employee benefit program under the control of the federal regulations stated in section 302(c) of the Labor Management Relations Act of 1947 or the ERISA act of 1974. The key parts of ERISA include fiduciary responsibility on the part of the employer; that is, assurance that plan assets are held in trust and that participants are informed about their benefits. What is important for providers of care/managed care organizations is that ERISA currently does not mandate any particular benefit design or provide for any particular arrangement in the provision of benefits. Therefore, the managed care organization/ providers that are contracting to provide care to employers under ERISA have much more latitude in developing the design of the benefit program and the contracting for the provision of those benefits to the enrollees of the program. Under current ERISA regulations a plan fiduciary is responsible for any loss resulting from the breach of the fiduciary's duty of care to the participants in the plan. If a managed care company/ provider organization accepts payment on a capitated basis, this fiduciary liability could extend to individuals who may provide health care determinations. Therefore, whether or not a participating provider to an ERISA plan is a fiduciary subject to liability is a question relating not only to the plan design but also to the activities of the provider under the plan. Because more and more employers have moved toward self-insurance, managed care organizations and their providers must be aware that under ERISA certain transactions and regulations prohibit self-dealing by a fiduciary. Depending on the provider's contract with either a managed care or a self-insured employer, the provider may wish to have competent legal advice as to the potential of self-dealing when a provider/organization controls or restricts services to a patient whereby it could be construed that the provider/organization will benefit from that action. *The whole area of ERISA regulations, as well as many other laws impacting physicians/ provider organizations, is a body of law that is changing and being interpreted differently from state to state, court to court, and year to year.* Those differences are another reason it is important to have appropriate and experienced health care legal counsel assist providers in moving into the area of capitated contracts.

Speaking of the potential problems with not providing services to patients under capitation, federal law prohibits HMOs contracting under Medicare/Medicaid from failing "substantially to provide an enrollee with required medically necessary items and services when the failure adversely affects or has the likelihood of adversely affecting the enrollee." This federal law, and some state laws that also prohibit providers from denying certain services, are the flip side of the main reason that federal and state governments, and many employers, are pushing and encouraging the move to managed care; for example, the need for providers to offer cost-effective and high-quality care. It is a given that to provide cost-effective care there is a need to control and minimize the cost of providing health care services to a defined patient population. Therefore, the efficiency of cost-effective care must be coupled with great attention to the quality and outcomes of that care.

We started this chapter with a mention of the long-standing concerns in health care relating to antitrust laws and the government's somewhat paradoxical application of them. The typical federal antitrust statutes used in relationship to the health care industry are the Sherman Antitrust Act, the Clayton Act, and the Robinson-Patman Act. Basically, these laws were passed by Congress long before managed care became a major part of health care delivery, and long before health care was anything but a cottage industry. Even so, these laws still are being applied by both the U.S. Department of Justice and the Federal Trade Commission to activities in managed care arrangements and organizations as well as in new forms of health care delivery. In general, the Sherman Antitrust Act prohibits contracts that restrain trade; for example, monopolies among competitors. The Clayton Act prohibits exclusive dealing arrangements such as mergers or combinations that may substantially lessen competition. The Robinson-Patman Act makes unlawful any price discrimination between competing or similarly situated purchasors where the effect may be to lessen competition.

Often times state antitrust laws parallel the federal laws. In other states, laws are also somewhat different and enforced differently by the elected attorneys general. Because of the differences from state to state, and because violations of antitrust laws can result in both civil and criminal penalties, I again recommend for physician networks negotiating managed care contracts that competent consultants and health care legal counsel be retained. Although it is not possible in one chapter to discuss all the legal issues relating to managed care and capitation, or even the antitrust issues such as price fixing, we point out that on September 27, 1994, the U.S. Department of Justice and the Federal Trade Commission issued statements of enforcement policy and principle relating to health care and antitrust. This would be a good place for physicians/medical groups and their legal counsel to start in determining the impact of antitrust laws on their particular managed care activity.

Another legal issue that is very state oriented is the corporate practice of medicine. In states that have passed corporate practice of medicine laws, a corporation may not practice medicine or employ a physician as its agent to practice medicine. This doctrine is based on the principle that businesses are not licensed by the states to practice medicine, only physicians. Certainly the relationship between a managed care organization and its physician providers needs to fit each individual state's corporate practice of medicine laws. This is particularly true relating to the degree of control by a managed care organization over the professional judgment of their providers and any conflict of interest arising between the physician and the patient attributable to the influence of a non-physician third party.

A similar issue related to the potential relationship between the managed care company and the provider is the variation from state to state relating to the ability or prohibition of a licensed professional dividing and sharing a professional fee or profit with another professional or non-licensed person.

Because of the Stark II laws, there has been a great deal of information in the public press and medical journals related to Medicare and Medicaid fraud and abuse. Basically Stark II laws prohibit paying for kickbacks for the referral of Medicare and Medicaid patients, as well submitting false claims to either Medicare or Medicaid. These federal and state laws need to be analyzed in each particular state where there is managed care and integrated delivery system activity. This is another body of law and regulation that seems to be changing fairly frequently. As an example, the federal government has developed and published various safe harbors relating to the anti-kickback aspects of Medicare. One such safe harbor addresses offering price reductions. Without going into any more detail, managed care contractual relationships need to be analyzed to ensure that the published safe harbors have been addressed and there is compliance with

areas like no payments for the referral of patients. This is particularly important because these laws provide for both criminal and
civil penalties, including substantial fines.

Lastly, one concern needs to be looked into when developing
a relationship for managed care purposes with an IRS tax-exempt
entity. Sometimes in the development of integrated delivery systems there is an assumption that by participation with an organization that is tax-exempt providers can benefit individually or collectively from the 501(c)(3) IRS status of a key hospital or medical
foundation as part of the delivery system. Realize that not only
may the nonprofit status of such an organization not be available
to individuals/medical groups but also unless the arrangement is
appropriately structured, the current tax-exempt entity may lose
its tax-exempt status. Contractual relationships with physicians
and medical group providers will definitely be scrutinized to determine whether or not the current tax-exempt status is going to
be appropriate for a new organization providing managed
care/capitated services in a competitive marketplace for a profit.
Certainly, physicians/medical groups need to be aware, as do the
tax-exempt organizations, that physicians/medical groups are
paying fair value for the services that they receive from a tax-exempt entity as part of their combined plan to deliver care in the
managed care arena.

These are only the highlights of the multitude of state and
federal laws and regulations that now impact physicians/med-
ical groups and their managed care partners and contracts. Like
areas of law impacting other industries, health care laws and regulations are likely to continue to change and have a changing impact on providers. This is particularly true for those
providers/medical groups that are going to be providing services under capitation in the future. Therefore, I close this chapter with the advice that physicians/medical groups continually
monitor their contracts from a legal standpoint. They and their
counsel need to determine whether any changes in state and federal laws since the contract was signed are now going to impact
the providers differently. As a reason for this caution, I refer
readers to the recent Marshfield Clinic, Marshfield, Wisconsin

case decided by a jury. This has impacted the Marshfield Clinic negatively for millions of dollars.[1] Since the financial impact can be substantial, the investment in appropriate consulting and legal advice in all of the areas mentioned earlier becomes a major part of successfully implementing capitated contracts.

CONCLUSION

Like the previous advice on legal issues for physicians and medical groups, I want to close this book with similar advice for all the issues and activities involved with making capitation profitable for physicians. By accepting capitated revenue and its associated financial risk, physicians/medical groups have changed their practice into a medical business. Physicians and medical groups can make such a medical business profitable. However, like any other for-profit business, to be financially successful at the end of the year requires a good product, good controls, good management, and good planning for the changes that will continue in the health care delivery business for years to come. Remember you can't drive successfully on the health care highway of the future by looking at the road in the rearview mirror. Making a profit with capitated contracts in the future requires a new way for most physicians to look at their practices, recognizing that negotiating and implementing appropriate manged care contracts will change their clinical and business practices.

---

[1]John McCally and Michel La Fond, "Marshfield Clinic Case," *CPA Health Niche Advisor,* Harcourt Brace Professional Publishing, December 1995.

APPENDIX

Managed Care Resources and Organizations

American Association of Physician-Hospital Organizations (AAPHO)—P.O. Box 4913, Glen Allen, VA 23058-4913.

American Association of Preferred Provider Organizations (AAPPO)—1101 Connecticut Avenue, Suite 700; Washington, D.C. 20036.

American Group Practice Association (AGPA)—Donald Fisher, Ph.D, Executive Vice President:1422 Duke St.; Alexandria, VA 22314-3930; (703) 838-0033.

American Health Information Management Association— Patricia Thierry, Chief Operating Officer; 919 N. Michigan Ave., Suite 1400; Chicago, IL 60611; (312) 787-2672.

American Hospital Association—

Donna Ganzer, Vice President; 1 N. Franklin St.; Chicago, IL 60606; (312) 422-3000.

American Managed Care and Review Association (AMCRA)— Charles Stellar, President; 1227 25th St. NW, Suite 610; Washington, D.C. 20037.

American Medical Association (AMA)—James Todd, M.D., Executive Vice President; 515 N. State St.; Chicago, IL 60610; (312) 464-5000.

American Medical Informatics Association—Jeanne Nevin, Acting Executive Director; 4915 St. Elmo Ave., Suite 401; Bethesda, MD 20814; (301) 657-1291.

American Medical Peer Review Association (AMPRA)—Andrew Webber, Executive Vice President; 810 1st St. N, Suite 410; Washington, D.C. 20002; (202) 728-0506.

Association of American Medical Colleges—Robert Petersdorf, M.D., President; 2450 N St. NW; Washington, D.C. 20037; (202) 828-0400.

Center for Consumer Healthcare Information—4000 Birch Street, Suite 112; Newport Beach, CA 92660; (800) 627-2244.

Center for Healthcare Information Management—Carla Smith, Executive Director; 3300 Washtenaw Ave., Suite 224; Ann Arbor, MI 48104; (313) 973-6116.

College of Healthcare Information Management Executives—Richard Correll, President; 3300 Washtenaw Ave., Suite 225; Ann Arbor, MI 48104; (313) 665-0000.

Computer-Based Patient Record Institute—Margret Amatayakul, Executive Director; 1000 E. Woodfield Road, Suite 102; Schaumburg, IL 60173; (708) 706-6746.

Federation of American Health Systems—Michael D. Bromberg, Executive Director; 1111 19th St. NW, Suite 402; Washington, D.C. 20036; (202) 833-3090.

Group Health Association of America, Inc; (GHAA)—Jane Fox, Vice President for Member Affairs; 1129 20th Street NW, Suite 600; Washington, D.C. 20036; (202) 778-3200.

Health Care Finance Administration (HCFA), Office of Managed Care—3-02-01 South Building, 7500 Security Boulevard; Baltimore, MD 21244-1850; (410) 786-3000; HMO Payment Mechanisms, (410) 786-1147.

Healthcare Financial Management Association—Richard Clarke, President; 2 Westbrook Corporate Center, Suite 700; Westchester, IL 60154; (708) 531-9600.

Healthcare Information and Management Systems Society—John Page, Executive Director; 230 E. Ohio St., Suite 600; Chicago, IL 60611; (312) 664-4467.

Healthcare Open Systems & Trials—Lewis Lorton, Executive Director; 444 N. Capitol St., Suite 414; Washington, D.C. 20001; (202) 434-4771.

Health Insurance Association of America—Bill Gradison, President; 1025 Connecticut Ave. NW, Suite 1200; Washington, D.C. 20036; (202) 833-3090.

Joint Commission on Accreditation of Healthcare Organizations—Dennis S. O'Leary, M.D., President; One Renaissance Blvd.; Oakbrook Terrace, IL 60181; (708) 916-5600.

Managed Health Care Association (MHCA)—A trade association of more than 120 major employers with an interest in managed care benefits. 1225 Eye Street NW, Suite 300; Washington, D.C. 20005.

Managed Care Consultants of America (MCCA)—John F. McCally, President; 45 Nord Circle; North Oaks, MN 55127; MCCAmer @ AOL.COM

Managed Care Information Center—3100 Highway 138; Wall Township, NJ 07719-1442; (800) 516-4343.

Medical Group Management Association—Frederick Wenzel, Executive Director; 104 Inverness Terrace East; Englewood, CO 80112; (303) 799-1111.

National Association of Health Data Organizations (NAHDO)—Mark Epstein, Executive Director; 254-B North Washington St.; Falls Church, VA 22046-4517; (703) 532-3282.

National Center for Health Statistics—6525 Belcrest Road, Hyattsville, MD 20782; (301) 436-8500.

National Coalition on Quality Assurance—200 L Street NW, Suite 500; Washington, D.C. 20036; (202) 955-3500.

National Committee for Quality Assurance (NCQA)—1350 New York Avenue, Suite 700; Washington, D.C. 20005.

Utilization Review Accreditation Commission (URAC)—1130 Connecticut Avenue NW, Suite 450; Washington, D.C. 20036.

G L O S S A R Y
of Key Managed Care and Contract Terms

Accreditation   Certification by a nongovernmental accrediting organization that a given health care provider or service entity meets that organization's standards; for example, the national Committee for Quality Assurance (NCQA) for managed care organizations, the Utilization Review Accreditation Commission (URAC) for utilization review organizations, the Joint Commission on Accreditation of Health Care Organizations (JCAHO) for certain health care facilities.

Accreditation Programs   As employers and other purchasers of health care increasingly become concerned with not only quality of care but also its affordability, an increasing number of provider organizations and health plans are going through accreditation programs to demonstrate their commitment to quality care and quality improvement.

Accrual   The amount of money that is set aside to cover expenses. The accrual is the plan's best estimate of what those expenses are, and (for medical expenses) is based on a combination of data from the authorization system, the claims system, the lag studies, and the plan's prior history.

Actuarial Assumptions   The assumptions that an actuary uses in calculating the expected costs and revenues of the plan. Examples include utilization rates, age and gender of enrollees, cost for medical services, and so on.

Actuary   A person who mathematically analyzes and prices the risks associated with providing insurance coverage, or who calculates the costs of providing future benefits. An actuary uses claims experience along with underlying costs, administrative expenses, and anticipated investment return.

Adjustable Premium   Usually used in connection with guaranteed renewable health policies in which the premium is subject to change based on classes of insured.

Adjusted Average per Capita Cost (AAPCC)   The Health Care Financing Administration's (HCFA's) best estimate of the amount of money it costs to care for Medicare recipients under fee-for-service Medicare in a given area.

Adjusted Community Rate (ACR)   A rate-setting methodology used by managed care plans to set rates based on expected use of health care services by a group. ACR includes the normal profit of a for-profit HMO or competitive medical plan. The ACR may be equal to or lower than the average payment rate, but can never exceed it.

Administrative Contract Services (ACS) or Administrative Services Only (ASO) Contract   A contract between an insurance company and a self-funded plan where the insurance company performs administrative services only and does not assume any risk. Services usually include claims processing, but may include other services such as actuarial analysis, utilization review, and so on.

Adverse Selection   Disproportionate enrollment into a plan by individuals with the potential for higher health services utilization than projected for an average population. An older population and impaired or chronically ill individuals are considered adverse risks. Adverse selection may cause premiums to be too low to cover actual plan experience.

Affiliated Service Group   A group of related companies, consisting of a service organization and other companies that have some degree of association and common ownership, that is treated as a single company for nondiscrimination purposes.

Age/Sex Rating   A method of structuring capitation payments based on enrollee/membership age and sex.

Agency for Health Care Policy and Research (AHCPR)   An agency of the U.S. Public Health Service, Department of Health & Human Services, that does scientific research, assessment of health care technologies, and support of clinical practice guideline development.

All-Payer Contract   An arrangement allowing for payment of health services delivered by a contracted provider regardless of product type (e.g., HMO, PPO, indemnity) or revenue source (e.g., premium or self-funded).

Allied Health Personnel   Specially trained and licensed (when necessary) health workers who perform tasks that may otherwise be performed by physicians, dentists, optometrists, podiatrists, and nurses. The term is sometimes synonymous with paramedic personnel, such as physician's assistants, or occupational, respiratory, and physical therapists.

Allowable Costs   Charge for services rendered or supplies furnished by a health provider that qualify as covered expenses.

Alternative Delivery System (ADS)   An alternative to the traditional fee-for-service health care system. ADSs integrate the financing of health care with providing patient care services. They may be in the form of an independent physicians association (IPA), health maintenance organization (HMO), preferred provider organization (PPO), or other managed care entity. Current trends have made these alternatives the norm in many urban markets. With insurers/payers moving toward prospective pricing methods (e.g., capitation), providers are adjusting to bearing greater risk and responsibility for appropriate resource allocation and usage.

Alternative Dispute Resolution (ADR)   Methods of resolving disputes, claims, and disagreements other than by the traditional legal system method.

Ambulatory Patient Group (APG)   An outpatient case-mix methodology that groups patient services and procedures on a weighted basis for purposes of fixing reimbursement.

Ambulatory Setting   An institutional health setting in which organized health services are provided on an outpatient basis, such as a surgery center, clinic, or other outpatient facility. Ambulatory care settings also may be mobile units of service, such as mobile mammography.

American Association of Physician-Hospital Organizations (AAPHO)   Established in 1993 as a resource of PHOs. Address: AAPHO, P.O. Box 4913, Glen Allen, VA 23058-4913.

American Association of Preferred Provider Organizations (AAPPO) A trade association of preferred provider organizations. Address: AAPPO; 1101 Connecticut Avenue, Suite 700; Washington, D.C. 20036.

American Managed Care and Review Association (AMCRA) A national trade association of managed care organizations such as HMOs, PPOs, individual practice associations, and utilization review organizations. Address: AMCRA; 1227 25th St. NW, Suite 610; Washington, D.C. 20037.

American Medical Peer Review Association (AMPRA) A national trade association representing federally designated professional and peer review organizations. Address: AMPRA; 810 First St. NE, Suite 410; Washington, D.C. 20002.

Ancillary Services The services performed prior to and/or secondary to a significant procedure, such as lab work, X-rays, and anesthesia; or a charge in addition to the copayment that the member is required to pay, such as to a pharmacy for a prescription that has been dispensed in nonconformance with the plan's maximum allowable cost list.

Antidumping Law A law that prohibits the transfer or discharge of patients for financial rather than medical reasons.

Antikickback Law Sometimes used to refer to the Medicare fraud and abuse laws that prohibit, among other things, paying or receiving kickbacks for referral of Medicare patients.

Any Willing Provider The laws in several states require any organization dealing with medical services to admit into the organization any provider that agrees to abide by the requirements of cost and quality.

Appropriateness Review A utilization management technique used by third-party payers under which individual cases are reviewed for clinical appropriateness and medical necessity of surgical and diagnostic procedures.

Arbitration A method of resolving disputes without use of the courts. A single arbitrator or panel of arbitrators is chosen by the parties to hear the case, and the parties agree to be bound by the arbitrator's decision. The arbitrator's decision is usually final; a court will not overrule it unless there was fraud or partiality involved.

Assignment A statement, usually included on a claim form, that permits the insured to authorize the insurance company or health plan to pay benefits directly to the provider of the services.

Balance Billing The practice of billing a covered person for the difference between the provider's fee and the usual, customary, and reasonable (UCR) fee covered by the payor. This may or may not be appropriate, depending on the contractual arrangements between the parties.

Base Capitation A stipulated dollar amount to cover the cost of health care per covered person, usually less mental health/substance abuse services, pharmacy, and administrative charges.

Basic Health Services   Benefits that all federally qualified HMOs must offer; defined under Subpart a, Section 110.102 of the federal HMO regulations.

Behavioral Health Care   Assessment and treatment of mental and/or psychoactive substance abuse disorders.

Beneficiary   Any person, either a subscriber or a dependent, eligible for service under a health plan contract.

Benefit Package   A collection of specific services or benefits covered by a managed care plan or insurance carrier.

Benefit Year   A 12-month period that a group uses to administer its employee fringe benefits program. A majority of subscribers use a January through December benefit year. A benefit year, however, may not match the fiscal year used by a group.

Best Clinical Practice   Best clinical practice is developed with the process of clinically identifying the most appropriate and effective care for a specific condition and continuous improvement on that care using feedback mechanisms such as clinical outcome research.

Billed Charges   A reimbursement arrangement under which fees for health care services are based on what the provider usually charges all patients for the particular services. Also called fee-for-service (FFS) reimbursement.

Board Certified   Physicians who have successfully taken the examination of a medical specialty board.

Board Eligible   Physicians who are eligible to take a specialty board examination as a result of completion of medical school and relevant residency.

Break-Even Point   The HMO membership level at which total revenues and total costs are equal and therefore produces neither a net gain nor loss from operations.

Bundled Billing   The practice of charging an all-inclusive package price or global fee for all medical services associated with selected procedures.

Cafeteria Plan   A flexible benefits plan, generally one that complies with the requirements of IRC Section 125 and offers a choice of two or more qualified benefits, or a choice between cash or one or more qualified benefits.

Capitation   A method of reimbursement where a health care organization receives a fixed per-member-per-month (PMPM) reimbursement for each of an employer's covered employees/dependents. The organization is then responsible for all medical services specified by contract for those members. Capitation can also be paid to certain specialists as a carve out payment for only that specialty's care for a given patient population.

Carrier   Refers to an insurance company, a prepaid health plan, or a government agency that underwrites and/or administers a range of health benefits programs including, sometimes, delivery of health care services.

Carve Out   Contracting separately for a service that is typically a part of an indemnity or HMO plan. Also sometimes referred to as single service plans (SSP).

Case Management   A process whereby covered persons with specific health care needs are identified and a plan is developed that uses health care resources to achieve the optimum patient outcome in the most efficient, cost effective manner. It typically integrates care provided by all the players—the payer, the provider, the patient, and the family—in an effort to find the most appropriate treatment for that person.

Case Mix   The relative frequency and intensity of hospital admissions or services reflecting different needs and uses of hospital resources. Case mix can be measured based on patients' diagnoses or the severity of their illnesses, the utilization of services, the characteristics of a hospital, or the various types of third party/private party payors for provider services to all the provider's patients

Cash Indemnity Benefits   Sums that are paid to insureds for covered services and that require submission of a filed claim. Insureds may assign such payments directly to providers of services (hospitals, physicians, etc.). Payments may or may not fully reimburse insureds for costs incurred.

Catchment Area   The geographic area from which an HMO/physician practice draws its patients.

Centers of Excellence (COE)   Health care facilities usually selected for specific services based on criteria such as experience, outcomes, quality, efficiency, and effectiveness.

Certificate of Authority (COA)   The state-issued operating license for an HMO.

Certificate of Coverage (COC)   A document provided to covered employees by the insurance carrier or managed care plan that outlines the benefits, covered services, and principal provision of the group health plan provided under contract by the insurer or managed care organization.

Certificate of Need (CON)   Usually a state requirement that a health care organization obtain permission from an oversight agency before making changes. Federally qualified HMOs are exempt from having to obtain a CON.

Civilian Health and Medical Program of the United States (CHAMPUS)   A health benefit program that provides coverage for armed forces personnel receiving care outside a military treatment facility.

Claims Services Only (CSO)   A CSO plan is a contract designed for fully self-insured employers that need very little administrative assistance. Under a CSO arrangement, the insurer administers only the claims portion of the plan.

Clinical/Critical Pathway Team   Clinical/Critical Pathway Team is a multidisciplinary team of generally 12 to 15 physician-directed, patient-centered caregivers. The pathway of care and care team activities are directed toward a single diagnosis or group of diagnoses. The team follows a common plan that helps to provide continuity of care and decreases in variances of care leading to quality improvement.

Clinical Practice Guidelines   Clinical practice guidelines are patient care guidelines and algorithms that describe a range of diagnostic and management strategies for a particular medical condition or group of conditions. Guidelines are intended for use by a broad range of health care practitioners, including primary care physicians, specialists, nurse practitioners and physician's assistants.

Closed Panel   The physicians whom members of a managed care plan are required to see because the plan has contracted with them to be on the panel; members cannot see physicians outside the panel of providers for routine care covered by the plan.

Coalition/cooperative/alliance/buying federation   A group of employers that organize to have an expanded employee base and combined purchasing power for negotiating better contracts with providers and insurers. This also gives the coalition/alliance leverage to negotiate for improved access to information relating to medical costs, quality, and better clinical outcomes.

Coinsurance   The portion of health care costs for which the covered person has a financial responsibility, usually according to a fixed percentage. Often coinsurance applies after first meeting a deductible requirement.

Collective Bargaining Agreement   An agreement between an employer and the bargaining representative of its employees.

Community Health Information Network (CHIN)   A system to electronically link providers, payers, employers, and consumers in communities to improve health care quality and promote community wellness.

Community Health Purchasing Alliance (CHPA)   A purchaser of health care benefits on behalf of employer groups.

Community Rating   Setting health insurance premiums based on the average cost of paying for services for all covered people in a geographical area, regardless of their individual history of (or potential for) using health services.

Comorbidity   Coexisting (usually chronic) conditions that may affect overall health and functional status beyond the effects of the condition under consideration.

Competitive Medical Plan (CMP)   A federal designation that allows a health plan to obtain eligibility to receive a Medicare Risk Contract without having to obtain qualification as an HMO. Requirements for eligibility are somewhat less restrictive than for an HMO.

Composite Rate   A uniform premium applicable to all eligibles in a subscriber group regardless of the number/age/sex of claimed dependents. The rate is common among labor unions and large employer groups and usually does not require any premium contribution by the union member or employee.

Concurrent Review   A utilization management technique used by managed care organizations to ensure that medically necessary and appropriate care is delivered to inpatients.

Consolidated Omnibus Budget Reconciliation Act (COBRA)   A federal law that, among other things, requires employers to offer continued health insurance coverage for a certain length of time to certain employees and their beneficiaries whose group health insurance coverage has been terminated.

Continuing Care Retirement Community (CCRC)   A community which, in exchange for an entrance fee and a monthly charge, guarantees lifetime housing and nursing care as required.

Continuous Improvement (CI)   Using quality indicators to achieve certain levels of patient care services.

Continuum of Care   A range of clinical services provided to an individual or group; this range may reflect treatment rendered during a single patient hospitalization or may include care for multiple conditions over a lifetime. The continuum provides a basis for analyzing quality, cost, and utilization over the long term.

Controlled Group   Two or more companies with a defined level of common ownership that are treated as a single company for coverage and nondiscrimination purposes.

Coordination of Benefits (COB)   A cost-control mechanism used by most insurers and managed care plans to avoid duplication of paying benefits when there is more than one insurance or managed care company responsible for payment of claims.

Copayment   A cost-sharing dollar amount that an insured person pays out-of-pocket for medical services. Copayments are used to discourage overutilization of medical services.

Cost Sharing   A general set of financing arrangements via deductibles, copays, and/or coinsurance in which a person covered by the health plan must pay some of the costs to receive care.

Cost-Effectiveness   The degree to which a service or a medical treatment meets a specified goal at an acceptable cost and level of quality.

Critical Pathways   Charts showing the key events that typically lead to the successful treatment of patients in a certain homogeneous population. They organize, sequence, and time the major interventions of nursing staff, physicians, and other departments for a particular case type, subset, or condition.

Current Procedural Terminology (CPT)   A list of medical service procedures performed by physicians and other providers. Each service and procedure is identified by its own unique 5-digit code. CPT has become one of the industry's standards for reporting of physician procedures and services, particularly to insurance/managed care companies for reimbursement.

Deductible   The up-front annual dollar amount that must be paid by the subscriber/member before insurance benefit coverage applies.

Dental Maintenance Organization (DMO)   A type of managed dental care plan that provides comprehensive dental services to enrollees for a fixed per capita fee, similar to an HMO, using a closed panel of dentists.

Dental Service Corporation (DSC)   A nonprofit organization that underwrites or administers contracts for managed dental care plans.

Dependents   Generally the spouse and children, as defined in a contract, of a person or subscriber covered by a health plan. Under some contracts, coverage may include parents and others.

Diagnosis Related Groups (DRGs)   A system used by Medicare for classification of inpatient hospital services based on principal diagnosis, secondary diagnosis, surgical procedures, age, sex, and presence of complications. This system of classification is used as a financing mechanism to reimburse hospitals and selected other providers for services rendered.

Direct Contracting   Individual employers or business coalitions contract directly with providers for health care services, often using a managed care company as a TPA. This enables the employer to include in the plan the specific services preferred by their employees at a rate controllable by the employer.

Disability   The inability to perform all or some portion of the duties of one's occupation or, alternatively, any occupation as a result of a physical or mental impairment.

Discharge Planning   A utilization management technique focusing on arranging for appropriate care after the patient is discharged from the hospital or other inpatient facility.

Disenrollment   The process of termination of coverage. Voluntary termination would include a member quitting because he or she simply wants out. Involuntary termination would include leaving the plan because of changing jobs.

Drug Formulary   A listing of prescription medications that are preferred for use by the health plan and that will be dispensed through participating pharmacies to covered persons. This list is subject to periodic review and modification by the health plan. A plan that has adopted an open or voluntary formulary allows coverage for both formulary and nonformulary medications. A plan that has adopted a closed, select, or mandatory formulary limits coverage to those drugs in the formulary.

Drug Utilization Review (DUR)   A quantitative evaluation of prescription drug use, physician prescribing patterns, or patient drug utilization to determine the appropriateness of drug therapy.

Dual Choice   Refers to the federal HMO regulation that requires employers who offer health insurance coverage to more than 25 employees to offer a federally qualified HMO plan as one of the health plan options.

Electronic Data Interchange (EDI)   The computer-to-computer exchange of business or other information between organizations. The data may be either in a standardized or proprietary format.

Eligible Individual   An employee who meets the terms and conditions established by an employer, or its designee, to participate in an existing health benefits plan.

Employee Assistance Program (EAP)   Services designed to assist employees, their family members, and employers in finding solutions for workplace and personal problems. Services may include assistance for family/marital concerns, legal or financial problems, elder care, child care, substance abuse, emotional/stress issues, violence in the workplace, sexual harassment, dealing with troubled employees, transition in the workplace, and other events that increase the rate of absenteeism or employee turnover, lower productivity, and other issues that impact an employer's financial success or employee relations management. EAPs also can provide the voluntary or mandatory access to behavioral health benefits through an integrated behavioral health program.

Employee Retirement Income Security Act (ERISA) A federal law enacted in 1974 that allows self-funded plans to avoid paying premium taxes or comply with state-mandated benefits, even when insurance companies and managed care plans must do so. This federal law governs almost all large nongovernmental employee benefits plans. Employers must comply with ERISA regulations if they self-insure the risks of their employee health benefits. Another provision requires that plans and insurance companies provide an Explanation of Benefits (EOB) statement to a member or covered insured in the event of a denial of a claim, explaining why a claim was denied and informing the individual of his or her rights of appeal.

Encounter Face-to-face meetings between a covered person and a health care provider where services are provided or rendered. The number of encounters per member year is calculated as the total number of encounters per year/total number of members per year.

End-Stage Renal Disease (ESRD) Terminal kidney disease. Sufferers are eligible for Medicare benefits.

Enrollee Any person eligible for services, either as a subscriber or a dependent, in accordance with a contract.

Episode of Care Treatment rendered in a defined time frame for a specific disease. Episodes provide a useful basis for analyzing quality, cost, and utilization patterns.

Exclusions Special conditions, such as preexisting conditions or circumstances, that are not covered in a group health plan.

Exclusive Provider Organization (EPO) A form of managed care plan, an EPO is similar to an HMO in that it can use primary care physicians as gatekeepers, often capitates specialty providers, has a limited provider panel, uses an authorization system. The main difference is that EPOs are generally regulated under insurance statutes rather than HMO regulations. Not allowed in many states that maintain EPOs are really HMOs.

Explanation of Benefits (EOB) Statement A statement mailed to a member or covered insured explaining how reimbursement was determined, why a claim was or was not paid, and the general appeal process.

Extended Care Facility An institution that provides skilled nursing, intermediate, or custodial care.

Favored Nations Discount A contractual agreement between a provider and a payer stating that the provider will automatically provide the payer with the best discount it provides anyone else.

Federal Employee Health Benefits Program (FEHBP) The program that provides health benefits to federal employees.

Federal Qualification The Health Maintenance Organization Act of 1973 encouraged the development of HMOs. Under this act, HMOs that voluntarily chose to comply with regulatory requirements more stringent than state law are eligible to receive federal grants and loans.

Fee-for-service   A traditional form of reimbursement in health care where total reimbursement is made on the basis of the number of services rendered to the patient. The risk of patient services lies with the insurers/payers.

Fee Maximum   The maximum amount a participating provider may be paid for a specific health care service provided to plan members under a specific contract. A comprehensive listing of fee maximums used to reimburse a physician and/or other provider on a fee-for-service basis is called a fee schedule.

Fee Schedule   A listing of accepted fees or established allowances for specified medical procedures. As used in health plans, it usually represents the maximum amounts the program will pay for the specified procedures.

First-Dollar Coverage   Feature of a health care plan in which the plan does not require its participants to pay any deductibles or copayments before benefits are received.

Fiscal Intermediary   An agency selected by HCFA to pay claims under Medicare, usually only one or two per state.

Flexible Benefits Plan (Flex Plan)   A plan that offers employees a choice among a number of alternative benefits.

Full-Time Equivalent (FTE)   The equivalent of one full-time employee. For example, two part-time employees are one-half FTE each for a total of one FTE.

Gatekeeper   A *primary care* physician or clinic responsible for all health care services provided to plan members. If plan members require the services of a specialist outside the primary care clinic, a specialist referral from the gatekeeper would be required.

Global Budgets   Federal and state government set funding amounts that are used as the baseline to make spending and reimbursement decisions. The fixed spending budget is used to cover all health care activities.

Global Fee   A method of setting payment rates on an all-inclusive basis.

Grievance Procedure   A formal process for the resolution of member or provider complaints, generally mandated by state law or federal qualification standards for HMOs.

Group Health Association of America, Inc. (GHAA)   A trade association for HMOs. Address: GHAA; 1129 20th Street NW, Suite 600; Washington, D.C. 20036.

Group Model HMO   A managed care model involving contracts with physicians in medical groups organized as a partnership, professional corporation, or other association. The health plan compensates the medical group for contracted services at a negotiated rate, and that group is responsible for compensating its physicians and contracting with hospitals for care of their patients.

Group Purchaser   A person or organization that purchases health care services on behalf of an identified group of persons, regardless of whether the costs of coverage or services are paid for by the purchaser or by the persons receiving coverage or services.

Group Without Walls (GWW)   A range of arrangements created to link physicians together by sharing central services, by forming a unit for contracting purposes, and yet having autonomy by keeping their own offices. Also known as clinics without walls.

Guidelines   Systematically developed statements on medical practice that assist a practitioner and a patient in making decisions about appropriate health care for specific medical conditions. Guidelines are frequently used to evaluate appropriateness and medical necessity of care. Terms used synonymously include practice parameters, standard treatment protocols, and clinical practice guidelines. Outcomes can be used as information to modify or improve guidelines.

Health Care Financing Administration (HCFA)   The federal agency responsible for administering Medicare and overseeing each state's administration of Medicaid. HCFA also manages HMO qualification and other utilization and quality review programs.

Health Care Quality Improvement Act of 1986 (HCQIA)   A federal regulation that affords antitrust immunity for good faith peer review activities. The reporting requirement is mandatory to the National Practitioner Data Bank (NPDB) for settlements and acts involving licensure and medical staff actions involving a physician's status.

Health Insuring Organization (HIO)   Usually an organization that contracts with a state or federal agency to assure the delivery of services to beneficiaries of a state or federal program such as Medicaid or Medicare. The HIO contracts with health services organizations, either on a discounted fee-for-service or a capitated basis, for the provision of hospital and physician services.

Health Maintenance Organization (HMO)   An organization responsible for providing or arranging the provision of comprehensive health care services, usually on a prepayment basis; for example, to enrolled persons within a designated population. Some HMOs emphasize prevention, wellness, and the gatekeeper model of primary care to maintain the health of their enrolled populations and lower costs.

Health Plan   The marketing/administrative organization of an insurance company or provider network of hospitals, doctors, clinics, and others, that provides a comprehensive range of health services.

Health Promotion and Prevention   Process of providing information, fostering awareness, influencing attitudes, and identifying alternatives so that individuals can make informed choices and change their behavior to achieve an optimum level of physical and mental health.

HEDIS 2.0/2.5   Health Plan Employers Data Information Set is a set of health plan performance measures that permits the trending of a specific health plan's data from year to year or comparison of measures among plans. Five major areas of performance are (1) quality of care, (2) access and patient satisfaction, (3) membership, (4) utilization, and (5) descriptive information on health plan management.

Hospice A facility and or outpatient service program that provides palliative care for the terminally ill by relieving pain and providing counseling; a physician may elect a hospice benefit in lieu of more active intervention. The facility is typically licensed, certified, or otherwise authorized pursuant to the law of jurisdiction in which services are received.

Hospital Affiliation A contractual relationship between a health plan and one or more hospitals whereby the hospital provides the inpatient services offered by the health plan.

Hybrid HMO Known as second-generation managed care systems, these organizations are extremely sophisticated in their organizational structures and product offerings. They tend to blur the differences among individual practice association (IPA) model HMOs, PPOs, and managed care fee-for-service indemnity health plans; hybrid HMOs offer open option or open ended products that modify the total lock-in of the traditional HMO enrollee to allow enrollees to use nonsystem providers but require a copayment, deductible, and so on. These offerings are also known as triple or multiple option products. The objective of such products is to allow the hybrid HMO to more effectively compete with PPOs and traditional insurance programs. This is similar to and sometimes called POS plan

Incentives As related to health services delivery, this term refers to economic incentives for hospitals by means of third-party reimbursement formulas to motivate efficiency in management or economic incentives for physicians who encourage decreased hospital utilization, promote judicious use of all resources, and increase delivery of preventive health services.

Incurred But Not Reported (IBNR) The amount of potential money that the plan or physicians may need to accrue to pay the claims for medical expenses from patients that have been referred elsewhere. These are potential medical expenses that the authorization system has not captured and for which claims have not yet been received. Unexpected IBNRs have been a major cause of financial insolvency for some managed care plans and providers.

Indemnify (Indemnification) Protection or security against damages or loss designed to make whole the one sustaining the loss.

Indemnity An insurance program in which the insured person is reimbursed for covered expenses.

Independent Living Program (ILP) A program of housing assistance, job retraining, and other types of assistance to help disabled individuals live as independently as possible.

Individual Practice Association (IPA) A health care model that contracts with an entity, which in turn contracts with physicians, to provide health care services in return for a negotiated fee. Physicians continue in their existing individual or group practices and are compensated on a per capita, fee schedule, or fee-for-service basis. Also called Independent Physician Association.

Integrated Delivery System (IDS) A generic term referring to a combination of providers to deliver health care in an integrated way.

Integrated Provider Network A network of physicians, hospitals, and affiliated providers combined for purposes of sharing clinical and financial risk, while providing a wide array of, or total, medical services.

International Classification of Diseases, 9th Edition (Clinical Modification) (ICD-9-CM) A listing of diagnoses and identifying codes used by physicians for reporting diagnoses of health care plan enrollees. The coding and terminology provide a uniform language that can accurately designate primary and secondary diagnoses and provide for reliable, consistent communications on claim forms.

Joint Commission on Accreditation of Healthcare Organizations (JCAHO) A private, not-for-profit organization that evaluates and accredits hospitals and other health care organizations providing home care, mental health care, ambulatory care, and long-term care services.

Length of Stay (LOS) The number of days that a covered person stayed in an inpatient facility. Average length of stay (ALOS) measures the average length of time a patient is in the hospital.

Long-Term Care Assistance and care for persons with chronic disabilities. Long-term care's goal is to help people with disabilities be as independent as possible; thus it is focused more on caring than on curing. Long-term care is needed by a person who requires help with the activities of daily living (ADLs) or who suffers from cognitive impairment.

Maintenance of Benefits (MOB) A type of coordination of benefits that limits the total reimbursement from all health plans to a given individual for a program of treatment.

Maintenance of Efforts (MOE) A requirement that employers increase benefits or provide refunds to Medicare primary employees to compensate for the reduced wraparound plan costs that resulted from the increased Medicare coverage of the Medicare Catastrophic Coverage Act.

Managed Care Form of health coverage where enrollee utilization patterns and provider service patterns are monitored before (prospectively), during (concurrently), and after (retrospectively) the actual delivery of services. Managed care usually has the insurer playing a much more active role in determining what is done for an enrollee, where it will be done, who will do it, and what they pay for it. Many businesses have determined managed care to be an effective mechanism in controlling their health care costs. Managed care entities can be designed in many ways; that is, as PPOs, HMOs, IPAs, or alternative delivery systems/integrated provider networks.

Managed Information System (MIS)   The common term for the computer hardware and software that provides the support for managing the plan, patient care services, and their costs by providers.

Management Service Organization (MSO)   A legal entity that provides practice management, administration, and support services to individual physicians or group practices. An MSO may be a direct subsidiary of a hospital or may be owned by investors.

Maximum Allowable Charge or Cost (MAC)   The maximum that a provider may charge for service. A related term, used in conjunction with professional fees, is *fee maximum.*

Medicaid   A health insurance program adopted in 1965 for eligible disabled and low-income persons and administered by the federal government and participating states. The program's costs are shared by the federal and state governments, and paid for by general tax revenue.

Medical Care Evaluation (MCE)   A component of a quality assurance program that looks at the process of medical care.

Medical Loss Ratio   The ratio between the cost to deliver medical care and the amount of money taken in by a health plan. The medical loss ratio is dependent on the amount paid for premiums as well as the cost of delivering care.

Medicare   A nationwide, federally administered health insurance program that covers the cost of hospitalization, medical care, and some related services for eligible persons, usually patients over 65 years old. Medicare has two parts: Part A covers inpatient costs. Medicare pays for pharmaceuticals provided in hospitals, but not for those provided in outpatient settings. Also called Supplementary Medical Insurance Program, Part B covers outpatient costs for Medicare patients.

Medicare Supplement Policy   A policy guaranteeing that a health plan will pay a policyholder's coinsurance, deductible, and copayments and will provide additional health plan or non-Medicare coverage for services up to a predefined benefit limit. In essence, the policy pays for the portion of the cost of services not covered by Medicare. Also called Medigap or Medicare Wrap.

Member Months   The total of all months that all members were covered in a given time period, usually 12 months per contract period.

Morbidity   An actuarial determination of the incidence and severity of sicknesses and accidents in a well-defined class or classes of persons.

Mortality   An actuarial determination of the death rate at each age as determined from prior experience. A mortality study shows the probability of death and survival at each age for a unit of population.

Network   An arrangement of several delivery points affiliated with a managed care organization; an arrangement of HMOs using one common insuring mechanism; a broker organization that arranges with physician groups, carriers, payer agencies, consumer groups, and others for services to be provided to enrollees.

Network Model HMO   An HMO type in which the HMO contracts with more than one physician group, and may contract with single and multispecialty groups. The physician may share in utilization savings, but does not necessarily provide care exclusively for HMO members.

Out-of-Pocket Maximum (OOP Maximum)   The maximum amount that an insured employee will have to pay for covered expenses under the plan.

Outcome Measurement   Outcome measurement is recording the outcomes/results of health care intervention. Measuring outcomes permits comparison to the original situation of the patient and is used for comparing outcomes of multiple physicians for the same patient problem/service.

Outcome Research   Outcome research is research that is designed to identify and analyze the outcomes and costs of alternative interventions for a given clinical condition to determine the most appropriate and cost-effective means to prevent, diagnose, treat, or manage the condition, or to develop and test methods for reducing variations in care.

Open Access (OA)   A self-referral arrangement allowing members to see participating providers for open panel specialty care without a referral from another doctor—typically found in an individual practice association HMO.

Open Enrollment Period   The period when an employee may change health plans. Usually occurs once per year. A general rule is that most managed care plans will have around half of their membership up for open enrollment in the fall, for an effective date of January 1. A special form of open enrollment is still law in some states. This yearly open enrollment requires an HMO to accept any individual applicant for coverage, regardless of health status, and only charge them the standard community rate. Such special open enrollments usually occur for one month each year.

Open Panel   A managed care plan that contracts with private physicians to deliver care in their own offices.

Out-of-Area Benefits   The scope of emergency benefits available to HMO members while temporarily outside their defined service areas. Some HMOs offer unlimited out-of-area emergency coverage. Others impose a stated maximum annual dollar benefit. Emergency coverage is usually the only HMO benefit in the total benefit package for which members may need to file claims forms for reimbursement of their out-of-pocket expenditures for care.

Outliers   A person who varies significantly from other patients in the same DRG/CPT code, such as a longer or shorter length of stay, death, or three times the average cost for a particular service.

Outpatient   A person who receives health care services without being admitted to a hospital.

Paid Claims   Measures what the carrier has paid, exclusive of employee cost sharing and provider discounts.

Part A   The portion of Medicare that covers expenses incurred in hospitals, extended care facilities, hospices, and so on.

Part B   The portion of Medicare that covers physicians' services and other types of care not covered under Part A.

Partial Disability   A disability that prevents an employee from performing one or more, but not necessarily all, material duties of his or her job.

Participating Provider   A provider who has contracted with the health plan to provide medical services to covered persons. The provider may be a hospital, pharmacy, other facility, or a physician who has contractually accepted the terms and conditions set forth by the health plan.

Patient Satisfaction Surveys   Patient satisfaction surveys are the scientific measurement of how patients feel about health care services and providers. The patient satisfaction survey now becomes a mainstream management tool for improvement and change in a health care delivery system. Techniques include nationally accepted surveys such as the Group Health Association of America's (GHAA's) protocol and survey form, monitoring of complaints, returns and customer service activities, focus groups, customer visits, warranty cards, standards, and indices.

Payer   Any individual or organization that pays for health care services including insurance companies and various government programs such as Medicare and Medicaid.

Peer Review   Evaluation of a physician's performance by other physicians, usually within the same geographic area and medical specialty.

Penetration   The percentage of business that an HMO is able to capture in a particular subscriber group or in the market area as a whole.

Per Diem Reimbursement   Reimbursement of an institution, usually a hospital, based on a set rate per day rather than on charges. Per diem reimbursement can be varied by service or be uniform regardless of the intensity of services.

Per Member Per Month (PMPM)   Specifically applies to a revenue paid to providers for each enrolled member each month.

Per Member Per Year (PMPY)   The same as PMPM, but based on a year.

Physician Hospital Organization (PHO)   A PHO is a legally recognized structure formed between hospitals and physicians. PHOs integrate the clinical, financial, and administrative functions of both entities. The premise is that the PHO will provide the full range of services for purchasers of health care in a more cost-effective manner.

Physician Profiling   Statistical comparisons of physician practice patterns regarding such things as numbers of visits, numbers of referrals, numbers of laboratory tests, and so on. The statistics are used to develop norms for identifying the most and least efficient providers.

Plan Administration   The management unit having responsibility to manage and control the health plan—includes accounting, billing, personnel, marketing, legal services, purchasing, possible underwriting, management information, facilities maintenance, and servicing of accounts.

Plan Sponsorship   The group that organizes the plan, finances its facilities, and/or makes up its governing board.

Point-of-Service (POS)   This product may also be called an open-ended HMO and offers a transition product incorporating features of both HMOs and PPOs. Beneficiaries are enrolled in an HMO, but have the option to go outside the network for an additional cost paid by the enrollee.

Policyholder   Under a group purchase plan, the policyholder is the employer, labor union, or trustee to whom a group contract is issued and in whose name a policy is written. In a plan contracting directly with the individual or family, the policyholder is the individual to whom the contract is issued.

Preadmission Review (PAR)   A utilization review mechanism used by plans that have telephone-based nurses review cases, assign expected lengths of stay, and issue authorization numbers.

Pre-Existing Condition (PEC)   Any medical condition that has been diagnosed or treated within a specified period immediately preceding the covered person's effective date of coverage.

Preferred Provider Arrangement (PPA)   Same as a PPO, but sometimes is used to refer to a somewhat less restrictive type of plan in which the payer makes the arrangement rather than the providers.

Preferred Provider Organization (PPO)   Term applied to a variety of contractual relationships between hospitals, physicians, insurers, employers, and/or third-party administrators. In a PPO, individual providers or organizations negotiate with group purchasers to make available health services for a defined population. This arrangement typically shares the following three characteristics: (1) a negotiated system of payment for services that may include discounts from usual charges or ceilings imposed on charges, per diems, or per discharge reimbursement; (2) financial incentives for individual subscribers (insureds) to use contracting providers, usually in the form of reduced copayments and deductibles, broader coverage of services, or simplified claims processing; and (3) an extensive utilization review program of provider services.

Premium   A prospectively determined rate that a member pays for specific health services. Generally, a comprehensive prepaid health plan has a premium rate established for single members and for families.

Preventive Health Services   Preventive health services have gained much attention over the last several years. Preventative service standards now require the development of specifications—clinical practice guidelines—for the use of preventive services, by most accreditation organizations.

Primary Care   Provision of basic or general health care by primary care physicians, nurse practitioners, physician's assistants, and other physician extenders. Primary care often emphasizes those medical services required to maintain good health or to treat simpler and more common diseases. Patients usually enter a medical care system when seeking primary care services and through a primary care gatekeeper physician in managed care situations.

Primary Care Physician (PCP)   A physician the majority of whose practice is devoted to internal medicine, family/general practice, and pediatrics.

Professional Review Organization (PRO)   A physician-sponsored organization charged with reviewing the services providing patients. The purpose of the review is to determine if the services rendered are medically necessary; provided in accordance with professional criteria, norms and standards; and provided in the appropriate setting.

Protocol (Algorithm)   A decision tree that describes a course of treatment or established practice patterns.

Provider   A physician, hospital, group practice, dentist, nursing home, home care agencies, pharmacy, or any individual or group of individuals that provides a health care service.

Quality   The features of a product or service that bear on its ability to satisfy the stated or implied needs of the user or consumer. Quality assessment usually includes consumers' evaluations of how well a product or service meets their needs and expectations with respect to process, outcomes, and perceived value.

Quality Assessment   Quality assessment stresses the importance of quality measurements as the basis for continuous improvement in a health care delivery system. Quality assessment addresses (1) quality assurance, (2) utilization management, (3) credentialing, (4) preventative health services, (5) rights and responsibilities, and (6) patient medical records.

Quality Assurance (QA)   A formal set of methods to measure quality of care.

Reasonable and Customary (R&C)   A term that refers to the commonly charged or prevailing fees for health services within a geographic area. A fee is considered to be reasonable if it falls within the parameters of the average or commonly charged fee for the particular service within that specific community.

Referral Provider   A provider (usually a specialty physician or other health entity) that renders a service to a patient who has been sent to him or her by a participating provider in the health plan.

Reinsurance   A type of protection purchased from insurance companies specializing in underwriting specific risks for a stipulated premium. Typical reinsurance risk coverages are (1) individual stop-loss, (2) aggregate stop-loss, (3) out-of-area, and (4) insolvency protection.

Reserves   A fiscal method of withholding a certain percentage of premiums to provide a fund for committed but undelivered health care and such uncertainties as higher hospital utilization levels than expected, overutilization of referrals, accidental catastrophes, and the like.

Residential Care Facility   A facility that provides adults with food, shelter, and some additional services.

Resource Based Relative Value Scale (RBRVS) A fee schedule introduced by the Health Care Financing Administration to reimburse physicians' Medicare fees based on the amount of time, resources, and expertise expended in selected specific medical procedures. Adjustments are made by regional variations in rents, wages, and other geographical differences. Developed by Dr. William Hsiao and a Harvard research team, it divides Medicare treatments into 7,000 procedures/services.

Respite Care Temporary care provided in a patient's home to give the primary caregiver time off from the demand of taking care of a family member.

Retrospective Review Determination of medical necessity and/or appropriate billing practice for services already rendered.

Return-to-Work Program A program of rehabilitation, job modification, and monitoring to get disabled employees back to work as soon as possible.

Rider A legal document that modifies or amends the coverage of a standard insurance policy.

Risk In insurance terms, it is the probability of financial loss associated with a given population. The term may apply to physicians, who may be held at risk if hospitalization rates exceed agreed-on thresholds. The sharing of risk by providers is often employed as a possible utilization control mechanism within the HMO setting.

Risk Management A program of activities designed to identify, evaluate, and take corrective action against risks of loss related to patient or employee injury, property damage, or financial loss from inappropriate or unapproved services.

Self-Insured The practice of an individual, group of individuals, employer, or organization assuming complete responsibility for the cost of medical expenses and other losses due to illness. Self-insurance is contrasted to the practice of purchasing insurance from a third party (an insurance company or managed care organization) by the payment of a premium to cover possible costs of receiving medical services and assuming the risk of medical service costs.

Severity of Illness A measure of the intensity or complexity of illness, often in conjunction with other preexisting conditions, usually estimated at the time of admission. It is used often when adjusting the outcomes of care to the sickness of the patient on admission. Some of the measures relate to the likelihood of death, some to loss or impairment of function, some to clinical efficiency of care (resources used per case), others to more abstract concepts.

Short-Term Disability (STD) A temporary period of disability usually not exceeding six months.

Skilled Nursing Facility (SNF) A facility that provides health and social services to patients on a less than acute basis when ongoing skilled care is required. These are commonly referred to as nursing homes.

Staff Model HMO A managed care model that employs physicians to provide health care to its members. All premiums and other revenues accrue to the HMO that compensates physicians by salary and incentive programs.

Standard Benefit Package A specified set of minimum medical benefits.

Stop-Loss Insurance   Insurance coverage taken out by a health plan/provider group or self-funded employer to provide protection from losses resulting from claims greater than a specific dollar amount per covered person per year, per illness

Sub-Acute   A level of institutional care for patients not requiring the intensity of services of a specialty or tertiary hospital but that typically support some services.

Subrogation   The contractual right of a health plan to recover payments made to a member for health care costs after that member has received such payment for damages in a legal action.

Subscriber   An employer, union, or association that contracts with an HMO for its prepaid health care plan, which is offered to eligible enrollees.

Superbill   A modified claim form that lists specific and/or specialty medical services provided by physicians. It does not substitute for claim forms required under most managed care plans.

Tertiary Care   Those health care services provided by highly specialized providers such as thoracic surgeons and intensive care units. These services often require highly sophisticated technologies and facilities.

Third-Party Administrator (TPA)   An independent person or corporate entity that handles group benefits, claims, and administration for a self-insured company or group. A TPA does not underwrite the risk.

Total Quality Management (TQM)   Total quality management is a new way of organizing/approaching the providing of services. TQM redefines quality by incorporating such factors as customers, suppliers, cost, continuous improvement, and price. Generally, total quality is a way of managing an organization that recognizes the customers/patients and the employees in adding value to the organization.

Triage   The classification according to severity of sick or injured persons to direct care and ensure the efficient use of medical and nursing staff and facilities.

Triple Option   Multiple option health care plans typically include indemnity, PPO, and HMO plans through one insurer. Triple option plans, in theory, prevent adverse selection by placing all employees in a single-risk pool.

Unbundling   Separately packaged units that might otherwise be packaged together. For claims processing, this includes providers billing separately for health care services that might be combined according to industry standards or commonly accepted coding practices.

Underwriting   Refers to bearing the risk for something; for example, a policy is underwritten by an insurance company. May also refer to the analysis of a group of patients that is done to determine rates, or to determine if the group should be offered coverage at all.

Uniform Billing Code of 1992 (UB-92) A revised version of the UB-82, a federal directive requiring hospitals to follow specific billing procedures, itemizing all services included and billed for on each invoice.

Uniform Clinical Data Set (UCDS) A computerized system to assist professional and peer review organizations in collecting medical record data and identifying cases with potential utilization or quality problems.

Union-Sponsored Plan A program of health benefits developed by a union. The union may operate the program directly or may contract for benefits. Funds to finance the benefits are usually paid from a welfare fund that receives its income from employer contributions, employer and union member contributions, or union members alone.

Utilization Management Utilization management is a keystone to effective health care management and is an important determination in both the cost and quality in a managed care organization. Appropriate utilization protocols and standards should be based on reasonable scientific evidence. Good utilization management systems monitor for underutilization as well as overutilization.

Utilization Review Accreditation Commission (URAC) An independent accreditation organization for utilization review organizations with a goal of encouraging effective and efficient UR processes and providing a method of evaluation and accreditation for UR programs. Address: URAC; 1130 Connecticut Avenue NW, Suite 450; Washington, D.C. 20036.

Waiting Period The period of time between an employee's hire and his or her enrollment in a health program.

Welfare Fund A fund into which employer and/or employee contributions for health care are placed and that is administered by a board, usually with equal representation from labor and management.

Withhold A percentage of payment to the provider held back by the HMO until the cost of referral or hospital services has been determined. Physicians exceeding the amount determined as appropriate by the HMO lose the amount held back. The amount of withhold returned depends on individual utilization by the physician; referral patterns through the year, groups of physicians, or the overall plan pool; and financial indicators for the overall capitated plan.

Workers' Compensation A state-governed system designed to address work-related injuries. Under the system, employers assume the cost of medical treatment and wage losses arising from a worker's job-related injury or disease, regardless of who is at fault. In return, employees give up the right to sue employers, even if injuries stem from employer negligence.

Wraparound Plan Commonly used to refer to insurance or health plan coverage for copays and deductibles that are not covered under a member's base plan. This is often used for Medicare.

INDEX

Administrative fee, 99
Adverse selection, 132
Antitrust, 161
Assignment, 88

Balance billing, 87
Bankruptcy, 68

Capitated medicine, 6
Capitation, 7, 37, 127
   base pay, 89
   distribution, 92
   dollar flow, 128
   expenses, 37
   incentive payment, 90
   incentive rates, 93
   payment distribution model, 115
   rates, 93, 110
   risks and rewards, 22
Clayton Act, 164
Clinic without walls, 11
Community rating
   flexibility, 111
   flexibility rating mechanisms, 111
   structures, 108
Composite index, 109
Continuum of care, 18
Contracts
   assignment, 69
   capitated contracts, 57
   capitation fund: PMPM, 74
   covered services, 75
   termination, 68
Coordination of benefits (COB, 58
Cost centers, 155, 156
   fixed costs, 156
   variable costs, 156
Cost data, 106
Cost effective care, 67
Cost target, 61
Counterproposal, 124
Covered service definitions, 106

Dependent, 58
Direct contracting, 7, 22

Economies of scale, 10
Electronic data interchange (EDI), 151
Employee Retirement Income
   Security Act of 1974 (ERISA), 162
   fiduciary, 163
   regulations, 163
Encounter form, 58
Evidence of coverage, 80

Federal Trade Commission, 164, 165
Fee for service medicine, 6, 127
Feedback information, 148
Financial modeling, 124
Financial risk, 162
Financial risk assessment, 123
   productivity, 123
   stop loss insurance, 123
   utilization, 123
501(c)(3) IRS status, 166

Geographic indexes, 114
Government compliance requirements, 83
Group practice evolution, 11
Group practice without walls (GPWW), 11, 12

HCFA contract, 81
Health maintenance organization (HMO)
   demographic factor, 109
   group model, 28, 29
   independent practice or physician
     association (IPA) model, 30
   market activity, 133
   market penetration, 4
   network model, 29–30
   PRO model, 31
   staff model, 27–29

HMO indexes
  inflation factors, 109
  premium rate structures, 109
Health Security Act, 4
Historical data, 159
Hospital ownership, 16
Hospital services, 58

Incentives salary incentives, 138
  salary plus incentives, 138
Income distribution model, 140–141, 144
  at risk withhold, 141, 143
  base salary, 140, 142
  case management credit, 142
  capitated income, 145
  distribution factors, 144
  patient service credit, 142
  performance credits, 140, 143
  prescription drug management, 142
  production credits, 140, 142
  seniority factor, 140, 142
  seniority split, 140
  utilization credits, 142
Incurred but not recorded (IBNR), 37, 150
Integrated delivery systems, 134, 135
Integrated group practices, 10

Legal concerns, 161
Legalese clause, 39
  appeals, 39
Liability insurance requirements, 67

Managed care
  defined, 2
  discounts, 22
  financial risk, 21
  five stages, 23–26
  medical director, 96
  performance indicators, 116
  primary care, 24
Managed care contracts, 33
  covered services, 36
  MCO medical director, 36
  per member per month (PMPM), 37
  risk sharing, 37
  subcontracts, 33
  termination, 39

Managed care organization, 51, 124
Management information systems (MIS),
    147, 149
  modeling, 149
  referral authorizations, 150
  what-if analysis process, 149
Management services organization (MSO),
    12, 134
Material default, 68
Medical director, 59
Medical foundation model, 16, 17, 18
  non-profit status, 18
  reserves, 16
Medical management fund, 61, 98
Medical services, 59
Medical services organization (MSO), 12
Medicare amendment, 80
Medicare, 81
  covered services, 81
  enrolled member, 64
  participating provider, 81
Medicare HMO 4, 5
Member, 59

Negotiation process, 51
Negotiation strategy, 51
Non-covered services, 64

Participating physician, 59
Per member maximum, 59
Per member per month (PMPM), 59, 92, 105
  capitation model, 112
  composite community rating factors,
      114
  premium rate model, 108
Physician agreement, 58
  amendment, 78
Physician income distribution, 137
  financial incentives, 137
  full risk contact, 137
  incentives, 137
Physician records procedures, 65
Physician reporting, 65
PHO (physician hospital organization), 5, 14
  closed panel relationship, 15
  opened panel relationship, 15
Practice activity, 41
PPO market penetration, 4

Preferred providers, 59, 64
Primary care (gatekeeper), 28, 130
Primary physician capitation, 59, 61
    covered services, 61
    distributions, 61

Rating mechanisms
    administrative and market expense
        flexibility, 114
    community rating by class, 114
    experience rating, 114
    family rates, 114
    geographic indexes, 114
    rates, 114
Referral patterns, 97
Referral services, 59
Referral specialists, 64
Reporting requirements, 66, 92
Resource management, 117
Risk adjust
    age/sex adjustment, 106
    risk-adjustment factor, 106
Risk assessment, 122
Risk contact
    analytical process, 104
    frequency, 107
    historical costs, 105
    utilization, 105

Risk/reward, 118
Robinson-Patman Act, 164

Service area, 59
Service exclusions, 106
Service standards, 67
Sherman Antitrust Act, 164
Stark II legislation, 139, 159, 161, 165
Stop loss, 129
Strategic analysis, 120
Subrogation, 59
Subscriber, 60
Subscription agreement, 60

Tail coverage, 68
Target number, 92
Total risk, 112

U.S. Department of Justice, 164
Utilization, 117
Utilization incentive monitoring, 117
Utilization review and quality assurance
    clause (UR/QA), 38, 65

Vertical integration model, 19
    decision-making process, 19

Negotiation, capitation, strategy, risk — today, these words are becoming as common as patient, hospital records, or primary care in most physician circles. This new terminology and its application are causing medical professionals to rapidly take notice and, willing or not, concede that managed care and capitation are here to stay. In fact, over 150 million Americans now receive their healthcare through managed care programs.

Physicians, trained in the clinical aspects of medicine and care of patients, are now expected to deliver not only quality care but also price and appropriate outcomes, all within the increasingly complex arena of managed care and capitated contracts. *Capitation for Physicians* addresses managed care's impact on physicians as the dominant mode of healthcare delivery and reimbursement in the United States today, equipping those physicians who are providing care with the information they need to have healthy practices as well as healthy patients.

Capitation for Physicians focuses on helping physicians and medical professionals understand the market-driven changes in today's healthcare delivery system. This hands-on guide offers providers practical information on how to understand, negotiate and implement a capitated contract for a successful medical practice. This includes:

- Understanding how to survive and be profitable in the changing managed care and capitated environment today.
- Improving negotiation and contract management skills.
- Providing the appropriate tools to stay on top of contract clauses and per member per month (PMPM) reimbursements.
- Cost-effectively implementing contracts by physicians and office staff.